T0218628

HEALTHCARE SUPPORT WORKERS

NHS support workers, such as nursing Healthcare Assistants, Maternity Support Workers, and Therapy Assistants, often provide the majority of face-to-face care to patients, clients and their families. This accessible guide explores the issues underpinning their recruitment, training, management, development and progression.

NHS support workers comprise four out of ten of the clinical workforce, yet despite their importance they have long faced barriers that mean they are not able to fully realise their potential. This is the first book to take a comprehensive look at this workforce, its history, the policy that shapes its recruitment, management and deployment, and explains clearly how their capacity and capability can be safely and effectively enhanced. Structured around the employment cycle, this text covers the introduction of Technical Levels, career changes, apprenticeships, recruitment and selection, informal learning, learning cultures, widening participation, supervision and functional skills. Providing practical, evidence-based guidance and including illustrative case studies, it suggests a range of interventions to overcome the long-standing barriers to the effective development and deployment of healthcare support workers.

Drawing on the latest research, and practice, including the author's own experience, this book is an important resource for all those educating, managing or recruiting unregistered healthcare practitioners. It will also provide invaluable guidance to healthcare support workers interested in progressing their careers.

Richard Griffin is Professor of Healthcare Management at King's Business School, King's College London. He has worked in NHS workforce policy for over twenty years. Richard has previously worked for the Chartered Society of Physiotherapy, the Department of Health and Social Care, and Health Education England. An author and co-author of over 200 reports, studies and articles, he was an advisor to the Cavendish Review, has undertaken extensive research into NHS clinical support roles and been involved, as an academic advisor, in national and regional workforce development programmes with both Health Education England and NHS England and Improvement. In 2015 he was awarded an MBE for services to health and social care.

HEALTHCARE SUPPORT WORKERS

A Practical Guide for Training and Development

Richard Griffin

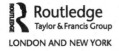

LONDON AND NEW YORK

Cover image: © Getty Images

First published 2023
by Routledge
4 Park Square, Milton Park, Abingdon, Oxon OX14 4RN

and by Routledge
605 Third Avenue, New York, NY 10158

Routledge is an imprint of the Taylor & Francis Group, an informa business

British Library Cataloguing-in-Publication Data
A catalogue record for this book is available from the British Library

Library of Congress Cataloging-in-Publication Data
Names: Griffin, Richard (Professor of healthcare management), author.
Title: Healthcare support workers : a practical guide for training and development / Richard Griffin.
Description: Milton Park, Abingdon, Oxon ; New York, NY : Routledge, 2023. | Includes bibliographical references and index. |
Identifiers: LCCN 2022009127 (print) | LCCN 2022009128 (ebook) | ISBN 9781032170596 (hardback) | ISBN 9781032170589 (paperback) | ISBN 9781003251620 (ebook)
Subjects: LCSH: Medical personnel. | Medical personnel–Training of. | National health services–Employees–Professional staff. | National health services–Personnel management.
Classification: LCC RA410.6 .G75 2023 (print) | LCC RA410.6 (ebook) | DDC 610.69071/55–dc23/eng/20220615
LC record available at https://lccn.loc.gov/2022009127
LC ebook record available at https://lccn.loc.gov/2022009128

ISBN: 978-1-032-17059-6 (hbk)
ISBN: 978-1-032-17058-9 (pbk)
ISBN: 978-1-003-25162-0 (ebk)

DOI: 10.4324/9781003251620

Typeset in Bembo
by Newgen Publishing UK

*For Anne without whom none of this would have been possible, and
Aleister, Emily and Molly for all your support and understanding. In memory of
my parents, Janet and Walter.*

CONTENTS

FIGURES

TABLES

BOXES

PREFACE

It is 2005. Tony Blair is Prime Minister. I had just been seconded from a Strategic Health Authority (SHA) in east London to work for the Department of Health in a new section that had just been established called the Widening Participation in Learning Strategy Unit. The Unit was headed by the late Professor Robert (Bob) Fryer who had been charged with seeing what the NHS needed to do to improve the education and development of its support workforce. We were based in an office block (now a smart hotel) between the Tate and Oxo Tower overlooking the Thames. Every morning I would look out of the window and marvel at the view.

Bob's task, with the Unit's support, was to produce a report for the Department of Health, which he did. It was called *Healthcare Learning for a Change*. The title, typical of Bob, was clever. On the one hand support staff struggled to access learning and it would mark a change if they could but also if they did it would lead to performance improvements. Throughout the report in meticulous detail, Bob set out the facts the Unit had gleaned about the NHS support workforce – that they had access to only a tiny proportion of the NHS's training budget and consequently struggled to acquire work-related qualifications, that the developmental initiatives that were provided for them were not sustained and that their contribution to care was not always valued, even though they were often the health workers in closest contact with patients. Bob would often remind us that 'the most vulnerable in our society, are cared for by the least trained, appreciated and paid members of the NHS workforce'.

Unfortunately, a change of prime minister meant that Bob's report was ignored, and the Unit wound up. My career took another turn, and I began working in Higher Education but focusing on healthcare support workers. My time in the Unit, and previously working for a Strategic Health Authority and the Chartered Society of Physiotherapy, had convinced me of the importance of the support workforce. It had though also shown me that they were under researched, under invested in, often under paid and frequently undervalued. In the words of Camilla Cavendish – the journalist who produced the next report on the support workforce and who I was an advisor too, support workers 'have been largely invisible to the public and policymakers' (2013: 83). The reasons for this invisibility and what to do about it are explored in this book.

I have had the privilege of working with many amazing people in NHS trusts, general practices, Integrated Care Systems, local authorities, trade unions and professional bodies, universities and colleges and arm's length bodies who 'get' the importance of support workers. Too often, though, great initiatives sit in isolation, are not sustained, or scaled. This means that whilst there are, as a senior midwife once told me, 'pockets of excellence' for many support workers the issues Bob Fryer identified two decades ago still apply. The good news is that things are changing for the better and all the pieces necessary to ensure support workers can maximise their contribution to care are in place.

My hope is that this book will help all those involved and interested in support worker recruitment, management, training, and development – healthcare students in further and higher education, support workers themselves, their managers and colleagues, heads of service, Human Resource and Workforce Departments, staff in arm's length bodies and ICS's, educators in independent training providers, colleges, and universities – put the pieces together so as to build support worker capacity and capability. In writing it I have drawn on research evidence and policy but also practice including my own experience and the experience of the many brilliant people I have been lucky to work with and for.

I hope more than anything that the book contributes to a greater understanding of this vital part of the NHS team.

Reference

Cavendish, C. (2013). Cavendish review. An independent enquiry into healthcare assistants and support workers in the NHS and social care settings. London, Department of Health. Available from: https://assets.publishing.service.gov.uk/government/uploads/system/uploads/attachment_data/file/236212/Cavendish_Review.pdf

ACKNOWLEDGEMENTS

None of us ever achieves anything alone and that is certainly true of this book. In the twenty years that I have been thinking about, researching and working with NHS support workers, I have been privileged to meet and be inspired by many great people. I have learnt from all of them, and many appear in the following pages. It would not be possible to list everybody here, but I would particularly like to thank: Dawn Grant, Professor Ian Kessler, Amanda Griffiths, Sue Johnson, June Mensah, Anita Esser, Claire Fordham, Professor David Sines CBE, Michael Wood, Denise Linay and Professor Bob Fryer, who sadly passed away in 2021.

For nearly a decade I worked with NHS employers in North West London. I would like to record my debt of gratitude to the workforce leads and other colleagues there who taught me so much: Alison Webster, Ralph Schafer, Goretti Downican-McAndrew, Sharon Probets, Maggie Orr, Liz Allibone, Pippa Nightingale, MBE, Kathryn Jones and Helen Parr. Further thanks are due to: Jessica Partington, Professor Karen Buckwell-Nutt, Ruth Auton, Sheryl Barnett, Ofrah Muflahi, Gita Malhotra, Lorraine Allchurch, Michelle Jenner, Gemma Hawtin, Jesse Manget, Kerry Mills, Suzanne Lilley, Marie Washbrook, Suraiya Hassan and Mary Somerville.

Finally, the merging of Health Education England (HEE) with NHS England was announced just as I completed this book. The HEE Talent for Care team, led by Kirk Lower, has done more than anyone in recent years to raise awareness of support workers in NHS and HEE occupation leads, particularly Bev Harden and Naomi McVey for AHPs, and Sally Ashton-May (for maternity), have developed strategies specifically aimed at upskilling and valuing the support workers. It has been a pleasure working with all of you.

Any errors or mistakes are mine alone.

ABBREVIATIONS

AHP	Allied Health Professions
APEL	Accreditation of Prior Experiential Learning
BAME	Black, Asian, and Minority Ethnic
BTEC	Business and Technology Education Council
CPD	Continuing Professional Development
FE	Further Education
FTE	Full Time Equivalent
GY	Grow Your Own
HASKE	Health and Society Knowledge Exchange
HCA	Healthcare Assistant
HE	Higher Education
HEE	Health Education England
HR	Human Resources
HRM	Human Resource Management
ITP	Independent Training Provider
KSF	Knowledge and Skills Framework
NHS	National Health Service
MSW	Maternity Support Worker
NVQ	National Vocational Qualification
RCN	Royal College of Nursing
RCM	Royal College of Midwives
RPL	Recognition of Prior Learning
RQF	Regulated Qualifications Framework
SEND	Special Education Needs and Disability
UCAS	Universities and Colleges Admissions Service

VET	Vocational Education and Training
WTE	Whole Time Equivalent
WDES	Universities and Colleges Admissions Service
WRES	Workforce Race Equality Standard

INTRODUCTION

The message of this book is a simple one: whether working in hospitals, general practice surgeries, clinics, domiciliary or in community settings, NHS clinical support workers, such as Healthcare Assistants, Maternity Support Workers, Therapy Assistants, Assistant Practitioners, Nursing Associates, Podiatry Assistants, or Physiotherapy Assistants, are a vital but neglected part of the NHS clinical workforce.

Support workers matter for a number of reasons.

Firstly, they comprise a significant proportion of the clinical workforce – almost 40%.

Secondly, in many settings, they are the healthcare worker who patients and their families have the most direct contact with. They provide a wide range of care and support, they deliver guidance and disseminate information and advice to people who are often in the most vulnerable periods of their life. They support patients who may be acutely or chronically ill or recovering from an injury or illness or suffering from a mental health condition or trying to improve their health and wellbeing. They perform a variety of tasks, from helping with personal hygiene, providing or taking information, motivating people to carry out exercises, setting up equipment, delivering public health programmes like smoking cessation, performing clinical tasks such as catherisation, positioning people before an X ray, recoding blood pressure, teaching parenting skills or correcting walking gait.

Benjamin Schneider (1987) famously wrote that organisations are the people that make them. This is probably more true of the NHS than any other organisation in the United Kingdom (UK) and as we have just seen support workers make up a significant part of the NHS workforce.

Finally, support workers matter because the NHS faces ever rising demand for its services; demand that will not be easily met unless the capacity and capability of

DOI: 10.4324/9781003251620-1

the support workforce is fully realised. Why that has not happened in the past and how to make it happen in the future is the subject of this book.

Important as this workforce is, the reality, until very recently, is it has been neglected (Cavendish, 2013 and Kessler et al., 2020). It has been neglected in terms of workforce policy, workforce planning, management, training, development, progression – and research. Support workers have rarely, for instance, been directly considered in Department of Health and Social Care policy documents. Nursing Associates aside, they do not feature explicitly in the workforce chapter of the *NHS Long Term Plan* (NHS England, 2019). When Health Education England (HEE) announced a £150 million increase in education funding in 2019 support workers were excluded (HEE, 2019). Arguably a workforce that already struggled to access 'consistent training' (Willis, 2015: 36), was not seen as important enough to receive support for their professional development. It is estimated that support staff, receive less than 3% of the NHS training budget (Kessler et al., 2019). As we will see in the following pages this neglect continues into the workplace, where support staff face an enduring set of barriers to their full deployment and career progression.

This workforce has also been neglected by the research community. A search of King's College London's databases of peer-reviewed journal articles with the word 'nursing' in their title, revealed 1,599,234 results. In contrast a meagre 3,821 results were generated when repeating the same search for 'Healthcare Assistant' and just two for 'NHS support workers'. Nursing Associates generated 435 results.[1] Although a crude measure this suggest that for every article about support workers, there are over 400 about registered nurses. Underlining this there is just one peer reviewed journal devoted to support workers – the *British Journal of Healthcare Assistants*. Many aspects of support worker's experience of working in the NHS have simply not been researched.

At first glance, then, a decade after Camilla Cavendish's (2013) review, it may appear that support workers remain, in the words of someone who has researched them, Carol Thornley (1997), invisible, and, sadly, for many this is the case. Long-standing barriers to their development and progression remain. Things are, though, beginning to change. In fact, support worker development is at a watershed. This is due, in part, to a growing recognition of the contribution they can make to care. This understanding was significantly heightened during the NHS's response to the Covid-19 pandemic. We are now seeing, for the first-time, specific strategies developed for support workers in a number of occupations as well as in 2020 a national campaign to promote and recruit people into support worker careers led by NHS England (2020). Change, though, is also happening because of wider government employment and skills policy that seeks to address long-standing shortfalls in Britain's vocational education system. Linked to this is a growing recognition of the NHS's role as a so-called 'anchor institution' in its communities and its ability, not least through its role as a major employer and commissioner of training to add social value (NHS England, 2019 and Health Foundation, 2021).

The need for this book

Given the growing recognition of the contribution that support workers can make to care and the need to consider more strategically their careers and deployment, coupled with the changes in the wider employment and skill landscape including NHS workforce planning operating models, it is timely to seek to provide a comprehensive overview of this workforce, one that embraces its recruitment, management, development and progression, as well as its history. There is no single book that brings together the latest research, policy and practice for *all* NHS clinical support workers to allow those who manage or teach or research or commission the services they work in and, most importantly, aspiring and actual support workers themselves, to maximise their contribution to safe and effective care.

This book seeks to fill that gap in a way that is both practitioner friendly and academically robust. It draws on research findings, insights and theory from a range of fields, including learning theory, the sociology of work, economics, labour market theory, employment relations and human resource management. This is the 'academically robust' bit, but I am always mindful that, as system theorist Myron Rogers (2017) has said, real change happens in real work and when people own the change that affects them.[2] I have, then, also tried to be 'practitioner friendly' in setting out information and guidance on interventions and processes that can be readily applied in 'real work'. Often, I draw on my own experience, working with others particularly in North West London (see Griffin, 2015 for a description of this work), to address the issues support workers can face.

How the book is structured

This book covers a lot of ground – schools' engagement, skills policy, local economic strategy, induction, Technical Levels, labour market interventions, workforce planning, careers, recruitment and selection, apprenticeships, diversity and equality, competences and pay and progression. In 2014 Health Education England (HEE) published *Talent for Care* – the first ever NHS workforce strategy solely focused on NHS support staff. *Talent for Care's* aspirations were organised under three headings – *Get In, Get Going* and *Go Further*.

With the addition of a fourth stage embracing pre-employment – *Get Ready*, this 'career journey' approach seems a sensible way to organise the discussion that follows. The support worker career journey begins before someone even decides to enter NHS employment by considering, for example, what factors influence people's choice of career and strategies for engaging with schools and colleges, as well as adult career changers. The importance of working with local labour markets will be stressed (all part of *Get Ready*). We will then progress to on-boarding – from recruitment to initial employment, including *The Care Certificate*. This is the *Get In* stage. We then move on to in-work development (*Get On*) and end with progression particularly into higher education (*Go Further*).

From an *employer's* perspective this career journey can be re-conceptualised in terms of Grow Your Own (GYO) workforce strategies. GYO focuses on local labour markets and the existing workforce as sources of capacity and capability and embraces approaches designed to bring people from outside the organisation into it (called *Outside/In* GYO), develop those in work (*In-work Development*) and also to support career progression (*Inside/Up*). Whilst treated as separate stages in this book there is a need for those responsible for workforce planning to recognise that GYO is a joined-up approach to workforce development that is 'end-to-end'. In a neglected review of the English vocational education system, undertaken in 2013 by Nigel Whitehead, then BAE Systems Group Manager, Whitehead makes the point that the system was fragmented, siloed and complicated. He pointed to the value of an end-to-end approach, as well as partnership working.

If you search on the internet for images of 'career journey' more often than not what you will see are pictures of staircases or ladders, suggesting that careers are always about moving upwards. Careers are rarely like that. They can be fragmented, turbulent and fluid (Hughes, 1959). This is particularly true for women and people in so-called lower status jobs (Kessler et al., 2019). Not every support worker wants to progress into registered grades: many want to do the best job they can in the role they are in (and they are a particularly loyal part of the NHS workforce) – and that is a good thing. However, taking a career journey approach allows a structured discussion of the distinct factors that shape the management and development of support staff at each stage.

What this book is not about

The focus of this book is the *NHS clinical* support workforce. Of course, every one of the 350 separate roles in the NHS matter, from porters to carpenters to finance staff to gardeners to receptionists. A book that tried to embrace all NHS support roles, their management and development would, though, be too long. One that also sought to encompass the equally important and larger still social care support workforce would be longer still and fail to do justice to these critical roles. In saying that my hope is that the insights and guidance presented in the following pages will be of value to non-clinical and non-NHS support workers and those concerned with their recruitment, management and development. Finally, the focus here is England, although references will be made to Scotland, Wales and Northern Ireland, where much good work has and continues to be undertaken in respect of support workers, but where health systems, structures and agencies differ.

Before anything else, though, we need to address the issue of how this workforce should be described. Like much in the world of support workers this is far from straightforward.

Nomenclature

The 'support' or 'assistant' – or as it was described in the past 'auxiliary', 'aide' or 'helper' – workforce is also sometimes described as 'untrained' or 'un-professional' or even 'unqualified'.[3] The workforce has also been defined in terms of its pay; as those NHS staff employed in *Agenda for Change* pay bands 2, 3 and 4. The *HEE Business Plan 2014–15* described 'Supporting health care assistants and **bands 1-4**' as one of its priorities (p. 21, emphasis added). Needless to say, registered staff were not described as 'bands 5-8' in this document. Other definitions have focused on the fact that the support workforce is not registered with regulatory bodies, such as the Nursing and Midwifery Council.

In fact all these terms used to describe the workforce – support worker, assistant, bands 2–4, unregistered, untrained, unqualified, unregulated – are problematical in as much as they define this large and important workforce in terms of either a deficit (lack of regulation, for example) or in terms of a subordinate relationship (to those they support or assist) or by their pay grade (a problem that registered staff can also face to be fair). This is an old problem. Writing about the nursing workforce in 1997, Edwards said: '"Unqualified" and "Untrained" have been accepted as synonymous adjectives by a profession that has demanded high quality preparation for its own members yet has been minimally involved in the development of its support workforce' (p. 243). In 1988 the United Kingdom Central Council for Nursing, Midwifery and Health Visiting defined support workers as a role that assisted nurses. Never mind that support workers frequently provide the bulk of hands-on care, and it could be argued should be fundamentally defined in terms of the assistance they provide patients.

There is another problem with these descriptions. They are not accurate. Whilst support workers are predominantly employed in *Agenda for Change* bands 2 to 4, some are graded higher. Whilst most are not registered with a regulatory body, some are. Voluntary registers exist and the Nursing Associate role is formally registered with the Nursing and Midwifery Council.

When discussing the clinical support workforce, I prefer a more expansive and positive definition.

I use the term 'support worker' to describe a diverse group of NHS staff that work in a wide variety of settings and occupational groups, often across organisational boundaries and agencies, providing direct care or support to service users of all ages including people receiving acute and critical care, seeking to change behaviours to improve their health and wellbeing and those with disabilities or mental health conditions. The tasks that support workers can perform could be clinical, technical, scientific or administrative and responsibilities vary from the routine to the complex. Support workers may work as part of a multidisciplinary team, or on their own or with an individual practitioner. The majority, but not all, are graded at *Agenda for Change* pay bands 2, 3 or 4. In educational terms their jobs require qualifications at education levels 2, 3, 4 and 5 although as with pay banding some support roles (such as physical exercise assistants working on rehabilitation pathways) may require higher level qualifications. In many settings they are the role that has the most direct contact with service users.

Given the richness and importance of the work undertaken by support workers, which the above paragraph gives just a glimpse of, describing them generically as 'support workers' as I do seems frankly to somewhat undersell them. It also begs a question we have already touched on, that Kessler and colleagues (2012) have raised: who do these staff actually support? Is it registered staff, service users or wider teams and groups? Kessler and colleagues concluded that, historically, they 'most obviously' have been framed in relation to the support they provide registered staff (ibid., 5). This was and is undoubtedly the case, but does this not diminish the contribution that support workers make to care directly themselves? As the role that often provides the most contact with service users, should that not be the main way the role is considered not in terms of the assistance they provide other staff?

This lack of clarity about the meaning of support work, vividly illustrated in the words used to describe it, stems from a lack of clear policy rationale for the expansion of the support workforce, which started in the 1990s. Rather than being seen in terms of an increase in capacity to care and support patients, the growth of the clinical support workforce was framed in terms of relieving the work of registered staff, or as a cheaper substitute for registered staff or as a stepping stone into registered grades, as much as a co-producer of care.

Nomenclature is problematical within individual occupations as well as more generally. Actually, that is a serious understatement. At least 21 titles are used to describe support workers employed in maternity services (Griffin, 2018) and a staggering 96 for support workers employed in mental health services (Nuffield Trust, 2021). Again, this is not a new problem. Support workers in nursing, historically, have 'been given a variety of titles including nursing auxiliaries, nursing assistants, ward orderlies, bath attendants and family aides' (Edwards, 1997: 238). This plethora of titles is once again the symptom of a lack of systematic national workforce planning which has resulted in decisions about titles (and entry-requirements, grading, roles and responsibilities) being taken by individual employers. Recommendations to standardise titles are in fact a common feature of the history of NHS support roles, starting at least as early as the Briggs Committee in 1972. Lord Willis (2015) is unlikely to be the last to call for an end of the 'profusion of titles' (p. 36).

As Leary and colleagues (2017) point out, following a review of the equally bewildering number of titles used to describe registered nurse specialist roles, variations in titles are confusing for patients, employers and those commissioners of services. In 1999 a former Health Minister, John Hutton, giving evidence to a health committee, admitted that support worker titles were not standardised and that these 'variations in job titles are not without significance. They are a testimony to the evolution of the role over a considerable period of time' (quoted in Kessler et al., 2012: 2). The fragmented development of support worker roles will be discussed in the next chapter.

This workforce though needs to be described, particularly if you are writing a book about them. So very much for the want of a better term I will use 'support worker' and 'support workforce' to describe this workforce collectively in the hope that there is consensus about a better term in the future – one that captures the contribution these staff make to care, the skills they bring and one that defines them in their own right. We have at least moved on from when support staff were formally described as 'helpers'.

Notes

1 Search undertaken: 20 September 2021.
2 Rogers (ibid.) saw systems as living and adapting rather than static. Another of his maxims was – connect as much of the system to itself as you can; an insight which is resonate in terms of vocational education and training and the need to collaborate with partners such as colleges, employment agencies and local authorities.
3 The headline of *The Telegraph* (Raynor, 2021) story about NHS funding on 9 September 2021 was: 'Nearly half of all NHS staff have no medical qualifications.' Support staff were described as unqualified assistants.

References

Briggs, A. (1972) Report of the Committee on Nursing, Cmnd. 5115, HMSO, London.

Cavendish, C. (2013). Cavendish review. An independent enquiry into healthcare assistants and support workers in the NHS and social care settings. London, Department of Health. Available from: https://assets.publishing.service.gov.uk/government/uploads/system/uploads/attachment_data/file/236212/Cavendish_Review.pdf

Edwards, M. (1997). The nursing aide: past and future necessity. *Journal of Advanced Nursing* 26, 237–245. DOI: 10.1046/j.1365-2648.1997.1997026237.x

Griffin, R. (2015). Building talent together. *Training Journal.* Available from: www.trainingjournal.com/articles/feature/building-talent-together

Griffin, R. (2018). *The deployment, education and development of maternity support workers in England. A scoping report to Health Education England.* RCM, Available from: www.rcm.org.uk/media/2347/the-deployment-education-and-development-of-maternity-support-workers-in-england.pdf

Health Foundation (2021). *Lifelong learning and levelling up: building blocks for good health. Why further education is critical to the levelling up agenda.* Available from: www.health.org.uk/publications/long-reads/lifelong-learning-and-levelling-up-building-blocks-for-good-health

HEE (2019). *Health Education England welcomes funding boost for 2020/21.* Available from: www.hee.nhs.uk/news-blogs-events/news/health-education-england-welcomes-funding-boost-202021

Hughes, E. (1959) The study of occupations. In Merton, R. and Broom, L. (eds), *Sociology Today,* Transaction Publishers, New York: Basic Books, reprinted in Hughes (1993), *The Sociological Eye,* London: Transaction.

Kessler, I. (2006). Strategic Approaches to Support Workers in the NHS. Pickett Institute and Said Business School.

Kessler, I., Heron, P. and Dopson, S. (2012). *The Modernisation of the Nursing Workforce: Valuing the Healthcare Assistant.* Oxford: Oxford University Press.

Kessler, I., Bach, S. and Nath, V. (2019). The construction of career aspirations amongst healthcare support workers: beyond the rational and the mundane? *Industrial Relations Journal* 50(2), 150–167.

Kessler, I., Bach, S., Griffin, R. and Grimshaw, D. (2020). *Fair care work. A post Covid-19 agenda for integrated employment relations in health and social care.* London, King's College London. Available from: www.kcl.ac.uk/business/assets/pdf/fair-care-work.pdf

Leary, A., Maclaine, K., Trevatt, P., Radford, M. and Punshon, G. (2017). Variation in job titles within the nursing workforce. *Journal of Clinical Nursing* 26 (23–24), 4945–4950. https://doi.org/10.1111/jocn.13985

Myron, R., quoted in NHS England (2017) *Leading large scale change: A practical guide.* Available from: www.england.nhs.uk/wp-content/uploads/2017/09/practical-guide-large-scale-change-april-2018-smll.pdf

NHS England (2019). *The NHS Long Term Plan.* Available from: www.longtermplan.nhs.uk

NHS England (2020). *Healthcare support worker programme.* Available from: www.england.nhs. uk/nursingmidwifery/healthcare-support-worker-programme/

Nuffield Trust (2021). *Untapped? Understanding the mental health clinical support workforce.* Nuffield Trust, available from: www.nuffieldtrust.org.uk/research/untapped-understand ing-the-mental-health-clinical-support

Raynor, G. (2021) Nearly half of NHS staff have no medical qualifications. www.telegraph. co.uk/news/2021/09/09/nearly-half-nhs-staff-have-no-medical-qualifications/, The Telegraph, 9 September 2021.

Schneider, B. (1987). The people make the place. *Personnel Psychology* 40(3), 437–453.

Thornley, C (1997) *The Invisible Workforce: An Investigation into Pay and Employment of Health Care Assistants in the NHS.* Unison, London

Willis, P. (2015). *Raising the Bar: Shape of Caring, A Review of the Future Education and Training of Registered Nurses and Care Assistants.* Available from: www.hee.nhs.uk/sites/default/files/ documents/2348-Shape-of-caring-review-FINAL.pdf

THE BASICS

Understanding education levels and credits

When you read a cookery book the first few pages are normally about the nuts and bolts of cooking: the equipment you need; the stock of basic ingredients; essential spices; oven temperatures; weight conversations and so on. Get this out of the way and you can get on with the much more interesting stuff of baking cakes. This section is the equivalent of that. The basics. Anyone with an interest in support worker recruitment, education and development needs to get to grips with the intricacies of the UK's formal education system. This can appear a little confusing and complicated, but actually is pretty straightforward. Honestly. The first step is understanding education levels.

The Regulated Qualifications Framework

Since 2015, in England, Wales and Northern Ireland, all formal education qualifications have been placed in a framework, called *The Regulated Qualifications Framework* (RQF). This comprises nine levels of increasing difficulty, ending at doctorates (PhDs). Grouped within each level are a varying number of different qualifications, each of which shares a similar degree of academic demand. This allows the multitude of qualifications that exist – and there are a lot of them – to be compared, although, because nothing in vocational education is ever simple, qualifications at each level may not actually be of equal value, because of their duration (see the discussion on Credits below). Table 0.1 sets out the seven RQF levels that are most relevant to support workers, along with a few examples of the qualifications within each.

Scotland also places its qualifications on a framework. This one is called the Scottish Credit and Qualifications Framework (SCQF) and comprises 12 levels, the first eight of which are relevant for support workers. Bachelor's degrees are placed on the SCQF at level 8.

DOI: 10.4324/9781003251620-2

TABLE 0.1 Education levels most applicable to support staff

Level	Examples of qualifications
Entry-level	Skills for Life, Entry-level diploma, Entry level English for foreign language speakers
1	GCSE 3,2,1 or D,E,F,G, Level 1 diploma
2	GCSE 9,8,7,6,5,4 or A*,A,B,C, Level 2 Certificate, Level 2 NVQ, Level 2 National Diploma
3	A Level, Level 3 Diploma, Technical Level
4	Certificate of Higher Education, Higher National Certificate, Level 4 Award
5	Foundation Degree, Higher National Diploma
6	Degree with honours

Apprenticeships contain RQF formal qualifications, such as diplomas and foundation degrees, and as such can also be placed on the RQF. For example, the *Healthcare Support Worker* apprenticeship is at RQF level 2, the *Senior Healthcare Support Worker* apprenticeship is at RQF level 3 and the *Healthcare Assistant Practitioner* apprenticeship is at RQF level 5. There are also apprenticeships at RQF level 4. For reasons I have never quite understood these different levels of apprenticeships also have their own categories, so that those at RQF level 2 are described as *Intermediate* apprenticeships, those at RQF level 3 as *Advanced,* those at RQF levels 4 and 5 as *Higher* and finally (and mirroring RQF language) those at RQF level 6 are described as *Degree* apprenticeships.

There are education and competency frameworks for a number of NHS support worker occupational groups. Potentially confusingly these also include 'levels' to distinguish different career stages. These do include RQF levels – as one of their aims is to standardise qualification requirements for support workers – but they also include competences, like communication skills which have different levels of demand. To avoid confusion, I will refer to 'RQF levels' whenever referring to a formal education. Oh yes, there are also different functional skills levels so that a RQF level 3 qualification is likely to provide the learner with a level 2 of functional skills (see below).

Credits

The relative position of a qualification on the RQF (or SCQF) describes its *comparative* difficulty in relation to a qualification at a different RQF level. 'Credits' refer to the *quantity* (size) of learning at any level. Ten hours of study equals one learning credit. Education programmes providing between one and 12 credits (i.e., between one and 12 hours of learning) are described as *Awards*, those providing between 12 and 36 credits are called *Certificates* and those providing 37 credits or more, *Diplomas*. An *Award, Credit* or *Diploma* is not restricted to any one RQF level. You can have a RQF level 1 *Diploma* as well as a RQF level 4 *Diploma*, for example.

Although at the same level on the RQF a RQF level 2 *Award* requires less learning (in terms of time spent studying) and therefore provides the learner with less credits than a RQF level 2 *Certificate*.

One more twist: credits are not the same as Universities and Colleges Admissions Service (UCAS) tariff points, which universities use to assess whether applicants meet their entry requirements (obviously because that would be far too straightforward!). Most qualifications, though, can be translated into tariffs. UCAS publishes an annual table showing the tariff points individual qualifications, including health related ones, are worth. The table for the 2022–23 academic year runs to a hefty 215 pages (UCAS, 2021). To take one example: the *City and Guilds Level 3 Diploma in Clinical Healthcare Support* is worth 65 credits (which is why it is a *Diploma*), which translates into 32 tariff points. By comparison the top A Level grade, also a RQF level 3 qualification, is worth 56 tariff points.

Functional skills

Being competent in English (the ability to read, write, speak and listen) and number skills (the ability to do calculations, record numbers, make and understand measurements and plan work) is an underpinning requirement of almost all education programmes, including those within apprenticeships. In fact, you cannot complete an apprenticeship unless you possess or obtain as part of the apprenticeship, the necessary functional skills. Functional skills also underpin safe and effective care by ensuring staff are able to, for example, communicate clearly with service users, record patient observations accurately and understand measurements, report an incident or follow a care plan.

There are three levels of functional skills attainment:

- Entry (1, 2 and 3)
- Level 1 (equivalent to GCSE grades 1–3)
- Level 2 (equivalent to GCSE grade 4 and above)

It is increasingly common, although by no means standard, that NHS employers ask for evidence of level 2 functional skills on, or soon after, employment but this is not mandated.

In addition to proficiency in English and number skills, NHS staff at all levels also need to be digitally confident and competent. As HEE state, digital skills are 'fundamental to the delivering of safe, effective and person-centred 21st Century care' (HEE, 2022). Digital skills include the ability to find and store digital data and use assistive technologies. As more learning is delivered virtually, digital skills are also important for staff wishing to study. HEE (2018) has produced *A Health and Care Digital Capabilities Framework* for all NHS staff based on six domains (each with six levels within them). The domains include Information, Data and Content, Digital Identity, Wellbeing, Safety and Security and Technical Proficiency.

English for speakers of other languages

There are many resources including training to assist people whose first language is not English, including some aimed specifically at staff employed in the NHS. Most adult education providers, such as colleges, deliver such programmes many of which are free.

Competency, competence and performance

It is worth being clear about some other terms too. Competency refers to the ability of someone to do something proficiently. In the context of healthcare that means having the knowledge (facts, awareness and understanding of something), skills (the ability to use the knowledge one has) and behaviours (the way someone acts particularly around others) to support service users. Competence, in this context, is what is deemed to be good practice. Performance is competency in practice (Chartered Society of Physiotherapy, 2020).

Conclusion

The best way I have heard the education system described is by imagining the RQF as a bookshelf. Each of its nine shelves contain books that are equally difficult to read. These are the levels. The next shelf's books are a little harder to read than the ones before and so on. The books on each shelf are not of equal length, however. *War and Peace* takes longer to read than *Catcher in the Rye* for example. The duration of study is measured in credits. I could stretch the metaphor by saying that the books on the RQF could also be fitted on a separate UCAS Tariffs bookshelf, which has been made bespoke to fit three or four A Level books! On top of all this there are functional skills, and everyone needs to have the right knowledge, skills and behaviours (competence) to perform their job effectively and safely.

Understanding this lays the foundations for the rest of the book.

References

Chartered Society of Physiotherapy (2020). Supervision, Accountability & Delegation. Information Paper. CSP. Available from: www.csp.org.uk/publications/supervision-acc ountability-delegation-activities-support-workers-guide-registered

HEE (2018). *A Health and Care Digital Capabilities Framework*. Available from: www.hee. nhs.uk/sites/default/files/documents/Digital%20Literacy%20Capability%20Framew ork%202018.pdf

HEE (2022). *Digital literacy of the wider workforce*. Available from: www.hee.nhs.uk/our-work/ digital-literacy

UCAS (2021). *UCAS Tariff tables. Tariff points for entry to higher education for the 2022–23 academic year*. UCAS, available from: www.ucas.com/files/tariff-tables

1

SETTING THE SCENE

Introduction

The management of human resources matters in all organisations, but this is arguably more the case in the NHS than most, if not all organisations where it can be literally a matter of life or death (Kessler, 2017). Healthcare is labour intensive and nearly four out of ten of the NHS workforce that provides direct care to patients are support workers. This chapter will describe what is known about that workforce, its career structure and history. The history of support workers, which is probably as long as the history of healthcare itself, is important because many of the challenges that support workers and their employers face are a product of that history.

The NHS support workforce

The NHS is the fifth largest employer in the world, after the United States and Chinese armed forces, Walmart and McDonalds, and the largest in the UK. It employs around 1.5 million people (Nuffield Trust, 2021a). In total one in every 25 working adults in England work for the health service and, of those, three-quarters are women (NHS England, 2019). This section describes the NHS clinical support workforce – its size, growth, composition and characteristics. This is not as straightforward a task as it should be. Much of the relevant data for this workforce is not gathered, meaning we need to draw on a variety of sources to try to understand it.

Table 1.1 shows the number (Full Time Equivalent (FTE) (see Box 1.1 below for descriptions of workforce measures), of clinical support staff employed in the NHS. For comparison this data is shown for 2009 and in 2021. In total 375,000 (FTE) support workers work in the NHS – an increase of 32% (26% for those support staff supporting doctors, nurses and midwives), since 2009. Nearly four

DOI: 10.4324/9781003251620-3

TABLE 1.1 The NHS Workforce (FTE)

Occupational group	September 2009	April 2021	Change (%)
Support to doctors, nurses & midwives	222,449	280,422	26.0
Ambulance support staff	12,926	24,842	92.2
Support to science & technical staff	48,594	69,908	43.8
Total support workforce	**283,970**	**375,172**	**32.1**
Total registered workforce (including doctors)	528,743	627,556	18.6
Total NHS workforce (including non-clinical staff)	1,002,298	1,195,431	19.2

Source: NHS Digital, 2021.

out of ten members of the NHS clinical workforce (37%) are support workers, a slightly higher proportion than in 2009 when it was 35%. Some caution needs to be taken in drawing conclusions about long-term trend as, over time, the size of the support workforce has ebbed and flowed. For example, Kessler and colleagues (2012) reviewed the relative growth in nursing and support staffing between 1995 and 2010 and found:

- Between 1995 and 2000 the number of support workers employed by the NHS grew and the number of registered nurses remained stable.
- Between 2001 and 2005 there was a steady growth in the number of support workers employed, but a steeper growth in nursing numbers.
- Between 2005 and 2008 support worker numbers remained stable but the number of nurses grew.
- Between 2008 and 2010 there was a slight growth in the numbers of support workers employed alongside a slight fall in the number of nurses.

Changes in the support workforce varies by occupational group. In mental health the Nuffield Trust (2021b) found between January 2010 and 2020 that the numbers of support staff *decreased* by 8%. It should also be remembered that the registered workforce is frequently subject to high vacancy rates. Despite the government's pledge to expand the nursing workforce by 50,000 staff, NHS trusts in 2021 experienced 37,000 vacancies (Ford, 2021).

In addition to the support staff employed in acute, mental health and community services, there are a further 6,657 clinical support workers working in general practices (Nuffield Trust, 2021a).

BOX 1.1 MEASURING STAFFING NUMBERS – DEFINITIONS

Headcount, sometimes described as 'Staff In Post', refers to the numbers of people working, at any time, in an organisation regardless of whether they are employed full or part time, on permanent contracts or temporary ones.

Full Time Equivalent (FTE) measures of workforce, also described as Whole Time Equivalent, take account of full- and part-time working, so that, for example, an employee working 18.75 hours a week, half the time of a full-time worker in the NHS, would count as 0.5 FTE but as 1.0 headcount. If a second person worked 18.75 hours, together they would count as 1.0 FTE (but 2.0 on headcount).

Funded Establishment (FE) refers to the number of posts that services are funded to employ. Difference between FE and FTE is accounted for by turnover and vacancy rates

Table 1.2 shows the proportion of Healthcare Assistants (HCA) employed in per 1,000 population. As can be seen, the UK is towards the bottom of the ranking with 1.4 HCAs employed per 1,000 population.

Workforce size aside, what else is known about the NHS support workforce? Drawing on the available research, Table 1.3 sets out details of the characteristics and composition of the workforce. Its diversity is discussed separately below. Discussing nursing support workers, Kessler and colleagues (2012) make the point, (which probably holds across all clinical occupations), that support staff 'have personal characteristics and life histories which distinguish them from qualified nurses and suggests that they bring distinctive capabilities and qualities to nursing care' (p. 2).

In common with the NHS workforce as a whole, the support workforce is 'highly feminized' (Kessler et al., 2016: 5, see also Thornley, 2007; Griffin, 2018; Nuffield, 2021b; and Kessler et al., 2021). Support workers are more likely to work part time than registered staff (Thornley, 2007 and Griffin, 2018), which may reflect the fact that they are also likely to also have caring responsibilities (Thornley, 2007; Kessler and Heron, 2007; Griffin, 2018; and Kessler et al., 2021a). Kessler and

TABLE 1.2 Proportion of HCAs: International comparison

Country	Proportion HCAs per 1,000
France	3.7
Lithuania	2.3
Czech Republic	2.0
Norway	1.8
Denmark	1.8
Switzerland	1.7
Canada	1.5
Japan	1.4
UK	**1.4**
Belgium	0.9
New Zealand	0.9

Source: Abboud and Neville (2021).

Heron (2007) describe support workers as typically 'mature women with domestic responsibilities' (p. 38). They are also more likely to have been recruited from their employer's local labour market (Kessler et al., 2016). Kessler and Heron (2007) found that many support workers had attended a school near to the hospital that they worked in. Once employed support workers are likely to remain loyal to their employer, more so than registered staff (Griffin, 2018; Nuffield Trust, 2021b). This may be a consequence again of them being recruited from local labour markets, and therefore already established in communities.

Many support workers – although not all – are likely to possess qualifications at RQF levels 2 and level 3 (Griffin, 2018, 2021). Data on the socio-economic background of the workforce is not known, although the evidence available, particularly education levels attainment, the fact that many are recruited from local labour markets and that many are sole or main earners in their household, suggests that they may be more likely to be from a different and lower social class than their registered colleagues. We will return to this in the next chapter when we consider dual labour markets.

The characteristics described in Table 1.3 seem to hold across pay bands and occupations. A survey (Kessler et al., 2021a) of Nursing Associates found that this workforce was predominantly female (91%), older (with 48% aged 35 years old or over), many Nursing Associates were the sole or main earner in their household and that 'on average respondents ... have worked in at least one non healthcare sector before joining the NHS' (ibid., 12). Although most had been recruited from the existing NHS workforce, a third had previously worked in retail and a quarter in the leisure and hospitality sectors. A national survey of Maternity Support Workers (Griffin, 2018) found this workforce to be overwhelmingly female (98%), with caring responsibilities (58%), working part time (55%) and more mature (56% were aged 40 years old or more) than registered staff.

The NHS produces comprehensive data on the ethnicity of its workforce by pay band (WRES, 2020). Table 1.4 sets out the proportion of the NHS workforce

TABLE 1.3 Characteristics of the NHS clinical support workforce

Characteristic	Source
Gender composition (female)	Thornley, 2007; Kessler et al., 2016; Griffin, 2018; Nuffield, 2021b; Kessler et al., 2021
Tend to work part time	Thornley, 2007; Griffin, 2018
Have caring responsibilities	Thornley, 2007; Kessler and Heron, 2007; Griffin, 2018; Kessler et al., 2021
Previous non-NHS employment and recruited from local labour market	Kessler et al., 2012; Kessler and Heron, 2007; Kessler et al., 2021
Loyal to NHS	Thornley, 2007; Kessler et al., 2016; Griffin, 2018; Nuffield, 2021b; Griffin, 2018; Kessler et al., 2021
Sole or main earner	Kessler et al., 2021

TABLE 1.4 Proportion NHS Staff by pay band who are BAME (2020)

Agenda for change band	% of NHS workforce who are BAME
1	19.5
2	18.3
3	16.6
4	15.5
5	27.5
6	18
7	15
8a	14.3
8b	11.9
8c	10.5
8d	8
9	8.4
Very Senior Managers	6.8

by *Agenda for Change* pay band who are from Black, Asian and Minority Ethnic (BAME) backgrounds. This data suggests that the diversity of the support workforce, defined as those employed in pay bands 1 to 4, is similar to registered grades, until the more senior grades (8b and above). Research by the Nuffield Trust (2021b) of the clinical mental health support workforce found that 27% of the workforce were male and that 14% were from BAME backgrounds. Kessler and colleagues (2021) found that one in ten of the Nursing Associates that they surveyed were from BAME backgrounds.

Kessler and colleagues (2016) described the support workforce, 'particularly in urban areas', as being 'ethnically diverse' (p. 5). This they suggest is a consequence of support staff being recruited from local labour markets and therefore being reflective of their community. This labour supply route could also mean, however, that in less ethnically diverse localities the support workforce may be less diverse an issue we will return too in discussing equality, diversity and inclusion in Chapter 5.

Support workers are the main 'bedside presence' on hospital wards providing the bulk of hands-on direct care and contact with patients (Thornley, 2007; Kessler et al., 2012; Cavendish, 2013; Willis, 2015; Kantaris et al., 2020; The Nuffield Trust, 2021b).

In summary, based on the evidence assembled, we can say that a 'typical' NHS clinical support worker is likely to be a woman, who has previously worked outside of the NHS before starting her healthcare career, most likely in the retail, leisure or hospitality sectors. She works part time, has caring responsibilities, is the main or sole earner in her household and lives near to where she works. She will spend more time in direct contact with patients than her registered colleagues. Finally, she is part of a workforce that is currently growing in size, although that has not always been the case.

NHS Support Worker Career Structure

Career structures matter, firstly, because they enable jobs to be appropriately designed and secondly, because they allow employees to see how they might develop their careers, helping them, and their managers, to make choices about development opportunities. The importance of career pathways in the NHS was stressed by *The NHS Long Term Plan* (NHS England, 2019), which pointed out that one of the reason people left employment was because 'they do not receive the development and career progression that they need. [Continuing Professional Development] – or more specifically workforce development – has the potential to deliver a high return on investment. It offers staff career progression that motivates them to stay within the NHS and, just as importantly, equips them with the skills to operate at advanced levels of professional practice and to meet patients' needs of the future' (p. 83). Whilst, not untypically, this comment was addressed only to registered staff (and not support workers), it does in fact apply to support workers equally. Indeed, lack of development opportunity is one of the reasons newly employed support workers leave and research shows that support workers, whilst aspiring to progress their careers, often do know how too (see Griffin, 2021 for example).

Clearly defined career structures also define scope of practice, support safe delegation of tasks and allow appropriate learning opportunities to be identified. One of the enduring issues the NHS support workforce has faced is a lack of consistency in terms of the tasks that they can and cannot perform. The roles and responsibilities of support workers have been left to the discretion of local employers. Career structures support consistency in job design and task allocation and ensure that the contribution of support workers is maximised. Implementation of the HEE (2019) *Maternity Support Worker Competency, Education and Career Development Framework* – the first official national attempt, in England, to define tasks for a group of support staff – increased capacity as services in a Local Maternity System ensured their support workers performed similar tasks (Griffin, 2019). For example, prior to the implementation of the *Framework* Maternity Support Workers (MSWs) in only one of the areas four NHS trusts undertook neonatal checks or checks for jaundice. Following implementation all did.[1]

Outside of primary care,[2] most support staff are employed in either NHS pay bands 2, 3 or 4, albeit with a small but growing number in band 5. In a straightforward sense for those support staff covered by *Agenda for Change,* these pay bands represent a career structure. New recruits could, for example, enter NHS employment at band 2, progress their careers to bands 3 and 4 jobs and then enter pre-registration healthcare degrees and progress into band 5 and beyond. Behind each pay band are *NHS Job Profiles,* based on the national job evaluation scheme (see Box 1.2 below). These seek to define, across most NHS jobs, roles and responsibilities and, in theory, should also support a career structure by setting out in a consistent way qualifications, tasks and competences expected at each band.

That is the theory. In reality, though *Job Profiles* are spartan in their descriptions. To take one example, the *Job Profile* for MSW roles has the following description in terms of patient's (sic) care. The *Job Profile* says the role 'Implements maternity care programmes, including providing advice' (NHS Employers, n.d.) Such vague descriptions lead to different interpretations of what a support worker employed in a maternity service may or may not do. Griffin (2018) explicitly sought to see whether there was a link between the tasks and responsibilities, MSWs performed and their grading and found that there was none. Identical clusters of tasks performed in neighbouring services resulted in different grading. Comparing job descriptions, The Nuffield Trust (2021b) found despite a commonality in tasks performed support workers employed in mental health services were particularly varied in terms of pay banding. There are also gaps in the *Job Profiles*. At the time of writing, there is no dedicated *Job Profile for* nursing support workers employed in mental health, for example.

BOX 1.2 NHS JOB EVALUATION AND *JOB PROFILES*

One of the aims of *Agenda for Change*, the NHS pay, and terms and conditions agreement introduced in December 2004, was to assure equal pay for work of equal value. Prior to *Agenda for Change* different NHS occupational groups' grading, terms and conditions were determined by separate agreements (this was called the Whitley system). *Agenda for Change* sought to bring most NHS staff under one national agreement (although medical staff and senior managers were excluded. *Agenda for Change* included a national job evaluation scheme.

Job evaluation seeks to break the components of a job down into distinct parts (which are called 'factors') and then assign points to these, with those factors deemed to be of particular importance allocated more points. This is called weighting. In the NHS scheme, the *Knowledge, Experience and Training* factor is judged to be more important than *Physical Effort*, meaning that, all other things being equal, a job requiring a masters-degree will score more highly (and therefore be graded more highly) than one requiring A levels or equivalent. To put it crudely, with job evaluation 'points mean prizes' – the higher the total score a job receives the higher it will be graded. Note that job evaluation assesses posts not people. An individual in a role requiring A levels may have a master's degree but this will not be considered under job evaluation because the post does not require it.

The NHS scheme has 13 factors: *Communications and Relationship Skills, Knowledge, Experience and Training, Analytical and Judgement Skills, Planning and Organisation, Physical Skills, Responsibility for Patient/Client Care, Responsibility for Policy and Service Development, Responsibility for Research and Development, Responsibility for Human Resources, Responsibility for Information resources, Freedom to Act* and *Physical Effort*.

So that every single job in the NHS did not have to be evaluated individually when *Agenda for* Change was introduced, national *Job Profiles* were developed setting out for each band 'typical' roles. These are used to compare actual jobs and determine their position on the *Agenda for Change* grading structure. In nursing there are *Job Profiles* for support workers at band 2 (called *Clinical Support Worker*), band 3 (also called *Clinical Support Worker!*) and band 4 (called *Assistant Practitioner/Nursery Nurse*). The *Job Profiles* suggest common titles for support workers within occupations but as the example from nursing shows these do not always address the nature of roles and do not seem to have led to greater consistency, as was discussed in the last chapter.

There have been periodic attempts to map out a career structure for support staff. An early example dating from 2010 was produced by Skills for Health. The sector skills authority designed a career framework for all NHS staff with nine levels (these are different to RQF levels and at the time there were nine *Agenda for Change* pay bands), four of which applied to support staff, with suggested titles and broad role and responsibility descriptions, as follows:

- Level 1 (called *Cadet*) at which staff require basic general knowledge and undertake a limited number of straightforward tasks under direct supervision.
- Level 2 (described as *Support Worker*). Staff at this level possess basic factual knowledge and may carry out a range of duties including clinical ones following set protocols, processes or systems.
- Level 3 (described as *Senior Healthcare Assistant/Technician*) staff have a knowledge of facts, principles, processes and general concepts in their field of work. They contribute to service development and carry out a wider range of tasks than staff at the Support Worker level below, but with supervision and guidance available.
- Level 4 (*Assistant/Associate Practitioner*) roles require factual and theoretical knowledge in their field of work. Whilst their work is guided by processes, protocols and systems, staff in level 4 roles exercise, within their scope of practice, their own judgement and plan activities.

In 2015 NHS Wales published *Developing Excellence in Healthcare. An NHS Wales Skills and Competence Framework for Healthcare Support Workers in Nursing and the Allied Health Professions.* This document aimed to provide 'a strategy for guiding and supporting career development' (p. 7). NHS Wales' *Framework* included education requirements and core competences linked to *National Occupational Standards* (see Box 1.3) and the *Knowledge and Skills Framework*[3] *Core Dimensions* (*Service Improvement, Health, Safety and Security, Personal and People Development* and *Communications*). More recently, NHS Education for Scotland produced its *Healthcare Support Worker Learning Framework* in 2020, which bought together a number of resources which 'values the contribution of [healthcare support workers] and promotes learning which will support safe and effective person-centred care' (p. 1). Professional bodies have also published competency standards or role and responsibility guide that include support roles (see Royal College of Midwives (RCM), 2011, for example).

BOX 1.3 NATIONAL OCCUPATIONAL STANDARDS (NOS)

NOS are nationally established standards of performance for work-based tasks and responsibilities across industries, including healthcare, with the underpinning knowledge requirements necessary for an individual to perform them proficiently. The NOS (2021) for undertaking an intravenous cannulation for example, which was developed by Skills for Health, comprises 22 separate performance criteria including an individual being able to 'access and accurately interpret all relevant work instructions and information' and 'maintain the cannulation site at regular intervals to avoid infection and maintain access' (p. 2). The 37 knowledge requirements underpinning this include an understanding of 'the clinical indications of infection in the insertion site' and 'the actions you would take if signs of infection are apparent and the implications of introducing fluids into the circulatory system when flushing cannula' (ibid., 5).

Whilst early attempts to define a career structure for clinical support workers had four levels, later developments reduced this to three stages. In part this reflected the ending of *Agenda for Change* pay band 1, but also an explicit move to incorporate RQF education levels into structures so as to standardise entry-level requirements. The framework HEE (2021) developed for AHP support staff, for example, has the following three levels:

1. At the first level roles are described as *Support Worker*. At this level staff use general skills and work under close supervision of registered staff carrying out straightforward clinical, technical, scientific and/or administrative tasks, for example performing housekeeping tasks, stock control or delegated clinical tasks. Fully trained staff at this level should possess a RQF level 2 qualification.
2. The next level's roles are described as *Senior Support Worker* and at this level staff use more advanced skills again under supervision, although they may work alone and directly deliver clinical, technical or scientific activities following training. Fully trained staff at this level should possess a RQF level 3 qualification.
3. The final level is called *Assistant Practitioner*. Staff at this level have in-depth knowledge and understanding about issues affecting health and well-being, possessing enhanced skills in their area of work, which could be a specialist clinical area. Fully trained Assistant Practitioners should possess a RQF level 4 or 5 qualification.

BOX 1.4 A NHS BAND 5 SUPPORT ROLE

There has always been scope for support roles to be graded above band 4 (so long as they meet the necessary job evaluation criteria), and not all posts at band 5 and above are regulated. An example of such a post is one held by Lorraine Allchurch from The Dudley Group NHS Foundation Trust where she works as Lead AHP support worker. Lorraine said that 'first and foremost I am a support worker with a clinical background as an Assistant Therapy Practitioner in Acute therapy services working across the disciplines of Occupational Therapy and Physiotherapy, Professional development has largely been targeted towards the registered workforce and this is where I see my role being pivotal to change that narrative. My aim is to provide opportunities and support staff to take these opportunities and be a voice for support workers. Meeting teams and hearing the views of AHP support workers has been a big part of getting this role established. Part of my current portfolio of work is, developing a "blended role" by providing enhanced training and competencies for clinical support workers to enable care to be delivered in a therapeutic manner. Working in collaboration with therapy and nursing teams to implement this role in some pilot wards to begin with. My vision for this role is to inspire and be a role model for AHP support workers, to not be limited or bound by titles, banding for your professional development, we can all have a meaningful contribution to the development of our roles and services we work within, given the right support and encouragement.'

We will return to the issue of career progression and structures in later chapters specifically in the context of the education and competency frameworks. As we have seen though there is currently no single consistent definition of the tasks and responsibilities support can – and cannot – perform. Why, given that support roles predate the creation of the NHS, is this the case? To understand the position of NHS support workers today, we need to understand their history.

A short history of healthcare support workers

Emergence: 1850s–1980s

For as long as there have been doctors, physiotherapists, nurses and midwives, there have been people assisting and supporting them and caring for patients. According to Stokes and Warden (2004) the term 'nursing aide' was first used during the Crimean War (1854–1856) to describe staff who assisted nurses care for patients (Kershaw, 1998). For the next century evidence of how these 'helpers' developed is slim. Edwards (1997) reports that the increasing professionalism of nursing in the later part of the nineteenth century, itself a response to the greater medicalisation of care, led to the establishment of training schools in many hospitals and consequently the existence of a trained nursing workforce, working alongside an untrained one. This untrained workforce grew in numbers during the First World War and were deployed supporting people in nursing homes with chronic conditions and in the care of the elderly (ibid.).

After the First World War where evidence does emerge about this workforce, it is mainly in the context of moves to close the nursing profession, for example when the General Nursing Council was established in 1919 and efforts were made to define the profession's scope of practice (Stokes and Warden, 2004), or in response to nursing shortages. On the eve of the Second World War, following concerns about a shortage of nurses, the Athlone committee was established under the Chief Medical Officer. One of the Committee's aims was to find additional staff to support nurses (Rafferty, 1996). The Committee noted that hospitals struggled to recruit sufficient numbers of both trained and untrained nursing staff (Edwards, 1997).

In 1955, just a few years after the creation of the NHS, the roles of 'nursing auxiliary' and 'nursing assistant' were formally recognised in the NHS grading structure (Stokes and Warden, 2004). Despite this formalisation of nursing support roles in the NHS grading system, there continued to be very little evidence of the tasks they performed during the 1950s, 1960s and 1970s or their experience of work. Kessler and colleagues describe 'the shape and nature' of the roles during these years as 'elusive' (2012: 22), but it appears, in nursing, that they performed routine tasks such as assisting patients with personal hygiene, along with housekeeping, clerical, and administrative tasks (ibid.).

The first explicit review of support roles, within the wider context of nursing workforce planning, was undertaken by the Briggs Committee on Nursing (1972). This noted the importance of nursing auxiliaries to services, but also found that half of this workforce had not received any training for their job, and a quarter of the remaining auxiliaries had just received induction training. Briggs thought that addressing the training needs of nursing support staff in a consistent way was a particular priority, although in a taste of what was to come, the Committee's recommendation was 'largely ignored' (Edwards, 1997: 241).

Briggs also considered the State Enrolled Nurse (SEN) role that had been created in 1961 and worked alongside registered nurses following completion of a two-year qualification. The report advocated that the use of SENs should be maximised but made no attempt to define the role, or the role of nursing support workers more generally. This was curious because Briggs did address the boundaries between nurses and other professions, such as AHPs, but yet was silent on where the boundaries between nurses and their support staff colleagues should be set (Kessler et al., 2012). As a result, according to Thornley (1996), 'nursing and non-nursing duties continued to be fluid and the role of experience vs formal training remained a point of contention' (p. 452).

The issues Briggs (op. cit.) raised in terms of nursing support worker access, or rather lack of access, to training continued to be an issue for this workforce into the 1980s. Edwards (1997), in her review of the available evidence, reported that all studies concluded that the NHS paid limited attention to the training needs of its support workforce and, as a result, support workers had limited access to learning, including in-house training. 'This lack of training has implications for the quality of care given to patients' (Edwards, 1997: 241). Edwards (ibid.) predicted that the number of nursing support staff employed in the NHS would grow due to shortages of nurses (a shortage which was at that point estimated to be 10,000) and rising demand for healthcare.

In fact, the actual number of support workers employed in the first four decades of the NHS rose and fell (Kershaw, 1998), with growth largely occurring in response to a shortage of registered staff – as was the case in physiotherapy, for example (Chartered Society of Physiotherapy, 2014). It was estimated that nursing auxiliaries comprised a not insignificant 25% of the nursing workforce (Meadows et al., 2000) and they have been described as forming 'a substantial part of the workforce' (Edwards, 1997: 237).

Outside of nursing, employees described as 'aides', began to be employed in physiotherapy and occupational therapy services soon after the Second World War. These roles performed largely housekeeping tasks and had little hands-on contact with patients. A shortage of physiotherapists in the 1960s resulted in a large-scale recruitment of aides, mainly from the existing nursing auxiliary workforce. The role was formally recognised as an official grade in the NHS Whitley pay system in 1973, being renamed 'remedial helpers' (Chartered Society of Physiotherapy, 2014).

The lack of evidence about the support workforce, including the work they undertook and impact they had on care, during this period is frustrating. Thornley (2007) comments on the 'negligible academic or policy attention…since [the nursing auxiliary's] inception despite the fact that much direct care was conducted by [the roles] and despite the importance of the roles' (p. 149). What can be said during this period is that support workers represented a significant proportion of the clinical workforce and that the issues they faced – unclear role boundaries and poor access to training – continue to this day. Issues that would become more pressing in the following two decades as a growing interest in support staff from policy makers, if not academics, emerged.

Growth: 1980s–2010

After being in the shadows for the first four decades since the creation of the NHS, the 1980s and 1990s saw a significant dedicated policy focus on the unregistered workforce by politicians, first in Conservative governments and then New Labour ones. Interest in the part support staff could play in delivering services, was mirrored in other parts of the public sector with, for instance, the introduction of the teaching assistant role in education. Although under different rubrics – New Public Management (NPM) in the case of the Conservative governments of this period (Clark, 2014) and 'modernisation' in the case of the New Labour governments of Tony Blair and Gordon Brown (Ferlie et al., 1996 and Falconer, 2005) – the focus on the support workforce was driven by common concerns about staff shortages, the need for greater management control, and increased marketisation as part of an efficiency agenda. In healthcare, workforce represents around two-thirds of total costs (Kessler, 2017), which particularly drove a policy interest in how efficiencies could be delivered through changes in skill mix (Kessler et al., 2012).

Project 2000 and the Health Care Assistant role

The first significant change for the NHS support workforce came as a result of *Project 2000* (Meadows et al., 2000). Published in 1986, *Project 2000; a Preparation to Practice* was produced by the United Kingdom Central Council for Nursing, Midwifery and Health Visiting, which was created in 1983 (later becoming the Nursing and Midwifery Council, sought to change the way registered nurses were educated. *Project 2000* resulted, amongst other things, in a stronger emphasis on academic study for aspiring nurses. In practice this meant student nurses spent less time on wards and more time in classrooms. This was significant because hospitals had previously made considerable use of students to help deliver care. This loss of capacity was supposed to be met through the creation of a new support worker role (Daykin and Clarke, 2000; Kessler et al.,, 2012) which was formally described as a *Health Care Assistant* (HCA) (Roberts, 1994; Daykin and Clarke, 2000).

Reactions to the introduction of HCAs at the time were ambivalent (Daykin and Clarke, 2000). The role was welcomed by many nurses and their professional body, The Royal College of Nursing (RCN), as a means of improving patient care (Roberts, 1994); however, concerns were expressed about the wider impact of the role. Whilst *Project 2000* could be framed as an attempt to address long-term problems of staffing shortages in nursing within the context of NPM, others saw the changes to nurse education and the introduction of the HCA role as a 'search for cheaper skill mix options' (Kessler et al., 2012: 23). Buchan, for instance, predicted that the introduction of HCAs, would result in support workers out numbering registered staff in nursing (quoted in Roberts, 1994) – despite the Department of Health, in 1996, stating it expected that HCAs should comprise no more than 11% of the nursing workforce (Meadows et al., 2000). Whilst the number of support workers did rise considerably over this period, they did not out-number nurses (Kessler et al., 2012). As it turned out, it was not registered nurses that HCAs replaced but rather the old nursing auxiliary role (Meadows et al., 2000) whose tasks they took over (Thornley, 2007). By 2010 only a 'rump' of nursing aides remained (Kessler and Heron, 2007). *Project 2000* also signalled the end of the SEN role. Some saw HCAs as a 'stalking horse' for local pay bargaining to the NHS (Meadows et al., 2000).

From the perspective of HCAs and their registered nurse colleagues, one area of contention was whether HCAs would receive sufficient training (Meadows et al., 2000). There was an 'expectation' nationally that HCAs would be attain a National Vocational Qualifications (NVQ) and also receive (in a foretaste of *The Care Certificate*), a three-month induction, however, due to training being determined by local employers' access was variable (Roberts, 1994, Daykin and Clarke, 2000; Thornley, 2007). One study found that just 30% of HCAs had acquired a NVQ by the end of the 1990s (Meadows et al., 2000).

Although a small-scale study based in a single NHS trust, Daykin and Clarke (2000) explored the attitudes of nurses and HCAs to the introduction of the role which, in this case, was an explicit attempt by the employer to change its skill mix ratio (between registered and unregistered nursing staff) from 60:40 to 51:49. Daykin and Clarke (ibid.) not only placed their study within the context of NPM, but also framed it in relation to attempts to close the nursing profession, then very much a live issue. They noted that determining the boundaries between HCAs and nurses was as important as determining boundaries between doctors and nurses. The concern, they suggested, might be that the 'use of healthcare assistants, instead of qualified nurses could be seen as undermining nurses' autonomy and professionalism' (p. 350). What they actually found was a more complex picture. Whilst nurses in the NHS trust they studied were indeed concerned that HCAs would erode their professionalism, including their holistic approach to care, the same nurses were, happy to give up tasks, particularly so-called 'dirty work', to HCAs. Kessler, Heron and Dopson (2015), in their exploration of the reasons why registered staff delegated tasks or not (which we will consider in more depth in Chapter 6), highlighted what they described as the nursing profession's 'dividend self', on the one hand wanting to horde all tasks and on the other wanting to discard some.

The HCAs, in Daykin and Clarke (2000) study, saw their role as 'offering valuable opportunities to develop knowledge and skills and achieve greater independence and job satisfaction' (ibid., 360), but were frustrated that the workload of their nursing colleagues meant their supervision and management were not prioritised.

In terms of the tasks that HCAs performed, Thornley (2007) reported that these typically comprised a range of general non-complex patient-facing activities such as bed making, patient observations, obtaining specimens, helping with catheter care, dressing and wound care (Thornley, 2007).

Despite the patient-facing nature of the role, Clarke (2014) found that the 'locally defined approach to HCA management excludes HCAs from management discussion leaving them virtually ignored as a group of workers' (p. 309). Thornley (2007), drawing on her research findings, in a similar vein, described the 'invisibility' of the HCA workforce (p. 149). More positively, there was other evidence showing that HCAs (many of whom had previously been employed in traditional nursing roles such as nursing auxiliaries), took the opportunity 'to develop their knowledge and skills' (Daykin and Clarke, 2000: 301) and that their contribution was valued by registered staff (Meadows et al., 2000).

Project 2000's recommendation that the title 'aide' should be used to describe all nursing support staff was not adopted.

New Labour, support workers and NHS modernisation

In May 1997 the New Labour government under Tony Blair was elected pledging to 'save' the NHS. Whilst NPM was a term coined by academics to describe a series of changes introduced in the 1980s, rather than an explicit and coherently articulated public policy by the previous Conservative administrations (Ferlie et al., 1996), the 'modernisation' agenda of the New Labour governments, particularly in health, was a much more clearly spelt out policy objective. Modernisation placed an emphasis on high quality public services delivered through performance standards, with an emphasis on the user rather than provider of services and partnership working with 'stakeholders' that could include the private sector (Falconer, 2005).

New Labour promised to increase spending on healthcare but also highlighted the need to modernise the NHS. As with NPM, this would have implications for support workers, as would the enduring shortages of professional staff and rising demand for healthcare (due to a growing and ageing population). In 2002, Derek Wanless published *Securing Our Future Health,* his report on the long-term funding needs of the NHS. Wanless explicitly mentioned the improvements that could be made by enhancing the role of NHS support workers. 'A significant change', he wrote, 'in the skill mix of the workforce is likely to be required, with a much greater role for Nurse Practitioners and health care assistants', although he acknowledged this 'would take time' (p. 91). There were, in fact, 22 mentions of 'skill mix' in his report.

In return for the increased funding the NHS received following acceptance of the Wanless (ibid.) report, there was an expectation that staff would work differently including the undertaking, by support workers, of tasks previously performed by registered staff (Department of Health, 2004; Kessler et al., 2012). This led to a raft of central initiatives although it is questionable whether collectively, they constituted a systematic strategy aimed at truly enhancing the contribution of support staff. As will be discussed, in the context of the tragic events at Mid Staffordshire and subsequent reviews, they did not seem to address long standing issues for support staff.

In 2004, the NHS Modernisation Agency, which had been set up in 2001 to assist delivery of reform in the NHS, published its *10 High Impact Changes Guide,* the last of which referred to workforce reforms, including the potential to make use of a new higher-level support worker role first developed in the North West of England called an Assistant Practitioner (see Box 1.5). Other policy developments aimed at the NHS support workforce introduced by the New Labour government, included individual Learning Accounts for in-work learning, which were introduced in April 2001, as part of *The NHS Plan's* (Department of Health, 2000) and New Labour's commitment to increase opportunities for staff without professional qualifications, the *NHS Career Framework* (Skills for Health, 2010) based on the new *Agenda for Change* grades, and the short-lived NHS University. The head of the NHS University, Professor Robert Fryer went on to produce, in 2006, the first official dedicated review of support workers in the NHS, in a report called *Learning for a Change in Healthcare* (Department of Health). Professor Fryer warned that the NHS did not take the learning needs of their lower graded staff seriously enough, with many struggling to access necessary learning including for functional (literacy and numeracy) skills.

BOX 1.5 ASSISTANT PRACTITIONERS

Assistant Practitioners were a role first introduced into the NHS in 2002 as part of New Labour's modernisation agenda, albeit with very little national guidance (Kessler and Nath, 2019). Assistant Practitioners are positioned (normally) at band 4 of *Agenda for Change*, just below newly qualified registered staff. They are (normally) recruited with a RQF level 3 qualification and then (normally) study a foundation degree (RQF level 5) which can be embedded within an apprenticeship standard. Practice, though, varies as Snaith and colleagues (2018) found in radiography where Assistant Practitioners in their survey possessed ten separate formal qualifications (some below RQF level 5). Reflecting this in their review of the history of the role, Kessler and Nath (2019) concluded 'knowledge and understanding of the assistant practitioner role in NHS England have long remained fragmentary and impressionistic, in large part a function of the roles nonregistered status and sensitivity to local circumstances' (p. 631). This lack of standardisation led Kessler and Spilsbury (2019) to describe the role as a 'malleable construct', a term that could be applied to support roles more generally.

Assistant Practitioners work in all areas of the NHS including primary care and across all clinical settings including on medical and surgical wards, care of the elderly, outpatients, theatres, maternity and radiography (Kessler and Nath, 2019). They deliver care to patients under the direction of registered staff but are able to work alone performing direct clinical tasks previously undertaken by registered staff (Skills for Health, 2009).

In 2017 Kessler and Nath (2019) surveyed 53 NHS trusts to gather information about Assistant Practitioner employment. Whilst half their sample employed 20 Assistant Practitioners or less (most frequently on medical or surgical wards), 22% employed more than 51. Two-thirds of Assistant Practitioners were recruited externally (with the remainder recruited exclusively from the existing workforce). The external recruitment of Assistant Practitioners suggested 'some maturity in the external labour market' (ibid., 629) the authors noted. The main reasons employers had introduced the role into their NHS trusts were, firstly, to support the provision of higher quality care, secondly, to retain existing support workers by creating an extended career structure and thirdly to relieve some of the workload of registered staff. At the time of the survey, just over half (53%) of the NHS trusts intended to increase the numbers they employed (13% expected to reduce the number), but the authors noted, this was before the extensive introduction of Nursing Associates.

Henshall and colleagues (2018) in a small-scale investigation of Assistant Practitioner roles found a lack of consistency in the role's deployment and confused boundaries between Assistant Practitioners and registered staff. They speculated that the Nursing Associate role would better define scope of practice, although, as will be discussed in Chapter 7, this may not be the case. For radiography, Halliday and colleagues (2020) found the 'assistant practitioner role...is not currently backed by a clear and consistent scope of practice that supports new opportunities for this area of the workforce' (p. 17).

Despite the emphasis on skill mix, new ways of working and the new Assistant Practitioner role, as in previous decades New Labour's modernisation agenda did not see changes in the proportion of support staff employed in the NHS. Actual numbers rose and fell during this period (Kessler et al., 2012). Deployment of support roles continued to vary by service with many struggling to access relevant education. The initiatives introduced by New Labour lacked sustainability, were not joined up or underpinned by a comprehensive strategy for NHS support workers.

BOX 1.6 THE DEVELOPMENT OF MATERNITY SUPPORT WORKERS IN THE NHS

Traditionally support workers employed in maternity services, as in nursing, performed housekeeping or clerical roles (Griffin et al., 2010). This began to change in England under New Labour, with the publication of the *National Services Framework for Children, Young People and Maternity Services* by the Department of Health (2004). This strategy envisioned a more expansive role for support workers in maternity services but the document did not provide extensive advice on what the roles could – and could not – do. In a rather short and conditional statement the *Framework* said that, once trained and working under the supervision of midwives, the role of a MSW 'could include infant feeding, advice and general information about the hospital environment' (p. 31).

In 2007 a new national maternity strategy, called *Maternity Matters* was produced by the Department of Health. This expanded the vision of the MSW role's scope slightly by adding 'parenting education' to the task list but again failed to clarify the full range of tasks the role could perform or the training it required. As a result, a series of evaluations of the role at the time, including by King's College London (2007), found a lack of adequate training and standardisation of duties. In response to the 'inconsistency and confusion about the tasks that support workers can perform' (RCM, 2011: 2) in England, the Royal College of Midwives (RCM) developed guidance on MSW roles and responsibilities. This did not though distinguish between grades but rather set out a full list of tasks that MSWs could and could not perform (following training and under supervision).

Despite the lack of attention by policy makers to the tasks that MSWs could perform, the value of the role was highlighted in the next national maternity review, undertaken by the National Maternity Review (2016) and called *Better*

Births. This strategy stressed the importance of MSWs in supporting maternity transformation, particularly in respect of public health, community postnatal care and intrapartum safety. To enable effective deployment of the role – and in recognition of its uneven development and deployment – HEE commissioned a review of MSW education and deployment (Griffin, 2018). The findings of this review, which identified a number of issues such as a plethora of job titles, inconsistent deployment (and consequently grading) along with limited access to training, led to the development of a dedicated MSW competency framework in England designed by University of West of England and an associated workforce strategy (HEE, 2019). Whilst welcoming the *Framework* the RCM remained 'concerned that the professionalism and loyalty of MSWs is often not rewarded by their pay banding and the opportunity to progress their careers' (Linay and Lloyd, 2020: 20). The framework (discussed in Chapter 5) is not mandatory, although there is evidence of the benefits associated with its implementation (Griffin, 2019).

Scotland took a different and more prescriptive and centralised approach by developing much earlier a national framework for the role (called Maternity Care Assistant (MCAs) and an associated education programme. The framework included an indicative job description that set out tasks and responsibilities. An evaluation by London South Bank University (2010) found MCAs had a positive impact on services. At the same time the role was also developed nationally in Northern Ireland and Wales.

The end of the New Labour government, in 2010, saw nursing become an all-graduate profession, something the profession had sought since at least 1919 (Stokes and Warden, 2004). Clark (2014) noted the significance of closure for the development of support worker roles, stating that during this period 'demarcation between nurses and HCAs [centred] on efforts towards occupational closure by registered nurses and a related division of labour between the two groups but one which is defined by registered nurses' (p. 301). In response to concerns that the move to an all-graduate profession would close work-based routes into nursing, The Department of Health published *Widening Participation into Pre-registration Nursing* in 2010. This set out the need for and benefits of work-based routes into the nursing profession, along with four models that could support existing staff progress, which took account of apprenticeships. The publication was one of the last healthcare strategies produced under a New Labour government. As we will see in Chapter 7, the issues it sought to address remain extant.

This period also saw profession bodies admit support workers into their membership for the first time. In September 1994, for example, staff graded as 'helpers' were 'encouraged' to join a separate list within the Chartered Society of Physiotherapy. Initially a qualified member had to nominate a helper to the list, but this restriction was dropped in 1997. In September 2000 the membership definition was loosened to allow rehabilitation assistants to join – reflecting the growth of 'blended' support roles that included elements, in this case, of physiotherapy and occupational therapy practice. In 2005 the term 'Assistant' was used to describe support workers in the profession. The Chartered Society of Physiotherapy now describes an Assistant as 'a person who is not a registered physiotherapist but is delivering physiotherapy or supporting the delivery of physiotherapy' (Chartered Society of Physiotherapy, 2014: 4). In 2001 the RCN created a category for support workers to join the professional body and in 2009 the RCM admitted MSWs, for the first time. Trade unions, like Unison, had always allowed support staff to join.

The number of support workers employed in the NHS continued to grow as the century turned, with the RCN (2007) reporting that numbers had doubled since 1997. In 1999 there were the first calls to regulate support staff. The Department of Health undertook a public consultation on regulating the wider workforce in 2004. Although the results of the consultation were never published, it showed that there was majority support for regulation of, at least, some support staff, such as Assistant Practitioners. There was also a recognition of the complexity of regulation. Ironically one aspect of that complexity was the lack of policy focus on the workforce which resulted in the absence of a national standardised qualification. Despite support from the RCN and a pilot in Scotland, however, regulation was not pursued (RCN, 2007).

Research continued to highlight that the issues support staff had long experienced such as uneven access to education, continued (Webb, 2011). Whilst policy makers were happy to advocate the increased use of support staff, they were less keen on tackling the issues that prevented the potential of this workforce to be fully realised.

Towards acceptance? 2010–2015

The attempts, albeit fragmented, to understand and increase the contribution of support workers from the 1980s, shone a light on the issues that the workforce faced. These issues would be bought into sharp focus following the events at Mid Staffordshire NHS Foundation Trust. Between 2005 and 2009 there were between 400 and 1200 deaths at the trust due to severe failures in care, such as a failure to provide patients with access to food or water. Sir Robert Francis was appointed by the government to publicly investigate the failings and his subsequent report made 290 recommendations, a number of which addressed support staff. He noted that the trust had experienced chronic staff shortages but also had failed to fundamentally care for its patients.

Francis (2013) made five key points in respect of nursing support workers. These were that they:

1. Provided the majority of direct patient care.
2. Were subject to little regulation.
3. Should be subject to registration before they practiced.

4. Should undertake standardised training including entry-level requirements.
5. Should have a common title such as 'nursing assistant'.

Writing at the time, the *Nursing Times* noted

> it is up to the ward or setting employing HCAs to decide how much experience and what qualifications they need. There are no minimum standards of training. Although the Nursing and Midwifery Council's code of conduct stipulates nurses must supervise junior staff, the [form this takes] depends largely on individual judgement. Mr Francis highlighted much of HCAs' work is unsupervised.
>
> *2013: 25*

The *Nursing Times* found that the vast majority of nurses (95%) supported the regulation of HCAs following the Francis report's publication (ibid.).

Initially the government's response to the recommendations, in respect of support workers, was to commission Skills for Health and Skills for Care to develop a code of conduct and standards of practice for support workers. The government also considered a voluntary register but rejected this as it was felt that standardised training would be too costly (see Chapter 6). Francis had though suggested that training costs could be covered by registration fees (op. cit.). The prime minister at the time, David Cameron, commissioned Camilla Cavendish, then a journalist at *The Times* and later to be head of Cameron's Policy Unit, to carry out a wide-ranging review investigating the issues nursing support workers in health and social care faced. Her report, along with Lord Willis's two years later, influenced the development of support workers in the NHS for the next decade and more.

The Cavendish Review

Camilla Cavendish was charged to investigated *nursing* support staff's recruitment, training, management, development and support 'to ensure that all those using services are treated with care and compassion' (2013: 85). She made seven key recommendations (most reinforcing Francis's (2013) recommendations) in response to the considerable barriers and issues she discovered many support workers faced, such as limited access to learning, multiple job titles and inconsistent deployment. Her main recommendations were:

1. All patient-facing support workers should complete a common certificate in fundamental care before they could care for patients.
2. Partly to assist progression into pre-registration healthcare degrees, but also to assist career development, a national Higher Certificate of Fundamental Care should be designed and made available to support workers.
3. All nursing support workers should be described as 'nursing assistants'.
4. The Nursing and Midwifery Council should make previous caring experience a pre-requisite for anyone joining a nursing degree.

5. Recruitment of support staff should focus on values and Directors of Nursing should play a more active part in the recruitment process.
6. A system of quality assurance should be developed for support worker training and qualifications so that funding was not wasted on ineffective courses.
7. The processes for managing poor performance should be reviewed. Francis (op. cit.) had made the point that support staff could be dismissed from employment at one NHS trust and begin working at another.

Talent for Care: The first NHS support worker strategy

In response to the Cavendish Review (op. cit.) the government called on HEE to work with employers to improve the capacity of the support workforce (HEE, 2013). A stakeholder group was established, and in October 2014 HEE published the NHS's first ever strategy concerned explicitly with support worker recruitment, education and development called *Talent for Care* (HEE, 2014a) and its associated *Widening Participation It Matters* (HEE, 2014b) policy. A national stakeholder group was established to oversee the implementation of the strategy and HEE staff in its regional offices given responsibility to oversee delivery.

Talent for Care (HEE, 2014a) clustered a series of recommendations, largely aimed at employers, around three key career stages, described as 'Get In', 'Get On' and 'Go Further'. The Get In recommendations sought to increase opportunities for people to enter NHS employment, particularly those from underrepresented groups through, for example, increased work experience opportunities and engagement with schools, colleges and local communities. Get On addressed the needs of staff in work, for example by advocating that all support workers had development plans and completed *The Care Certificate*. Finally, Go Further was concerned with career progression including into pre-registration degrees. A related school's engagement strategy was also published to support Get In (HEE, nd). It should be noted that although Cavendish focused on the nursing support workforce, *Talent for Care* covered all NHS clinical support roles.

A stakeholder group that HEE established created a new standards-based induction programme, called *The Care Certificate,* discussed in Chapter 4, for all patient facing NHS support staff. Cavendish's proposal for a higher care certificate was not pursued nationally. *The Care Certificate* was, in fact, the only recommendation made by Cavendish (op. cit.), or indeed Francis (op. cit.) that was fully backed by government. Whether employers implemented the new HEE (2014a, 2014b and n.d.) strategies, such as seeking to recruit underrepresented groups, was left to their discretion.

Two years after the publication of *Talent for Care* (op. cit.), an evaluation of the strategy comprising a survey of 120 employers along with case studies, was undertaken by King's College London to assess its effectiveness (Kessler et al., 2016). This uncovered a mixed picture. Whilst half of survey respondents reported that their NHS trust board had considered the strategy and a third felt that it had increased the profile of support staff within their organisation, investment in support worker education remained very low (estimated by the researchers at 3% of total training funds), and the majority of respondents doubted whether there was sufficient capacity in their organisation to implement the full proposals. Moreover, two-thirds of the employers sampled felt that the strategy only reflected work that they were already doing. A few years later Griffin (2018) found that only 5% of MSWs had heard of *Talent for Care*.

Talent for Care (op. cit.) was subsequently, in the words of HEE 'extended to staff at all levels' (HEE, 2021b). It is unclear whether the strategy is increasingly of historic interest or will again act as a focus for support worker development.

The Shape of Caring *review*

Two years after the publication of the Cavendish Review (op. cit.), HEE, in partnership with the Nursing and Midwifery Council, commissioned a review of nurse education that included nursing support staff. *The Shape of Caring*, headed by Lord Willis, was published in February 2015. It made 34 recommendations in respect of nursing education and training. Lord Willis devoted a chapter to nursing support worker roles, noting, like those before him, that they frequently provided the majority of hands-on care and experienced a by now familiar set of issues. 'Care assistants', Willis wrote, 'have no compulsory or consistent training and operate with a profusion of job titles' (2015: 36). *The Shape of Caring* made a series of recommendations, most reiterating previous reviews:

- The Higher Care Certificate, as well as The Care Certificate, should be implemented.
- Common competency standards should be developed.
- There should be national job descriptions and role titles.
- A new band 3 role should be created that 'would act as a bridge between unregulated care assistant workforce and the registered workforce' (Willis, 2015: 39).
- Universities should recognise prior experience when considering applications for nursing degree programmes.
- Workplace routes into degrees should be created.
- Support staff should have e-portfolios and skills passports.

The only recommendation that was actually enacted was the proposal to create a new 'bridging' role, although rather than at band 3 as Willis recommended, the Nursing Associate was created at band 4 (see Chapter 7).

Conclusion

Looking back at the long history of support workers covered in this chapter, two things stick out.

The first is the extent to which the workforce has been neglected. Very little is known about their numbers or the tasks that they performed, certainly up to the 1990s. There is minimal research on the roles, their impact or support workers experience of working in healthcare. It was only in the closing decades of the last century that they were allowed to join professional bodies.

The second issue is the absence of a substantive strategy underpinning the roles. There have been a number of initiatives aimed at their management and development, but most were not sustained, such as Learning Accounts or the NHS University, or joined up. Consequently, there is no consistent systematic discourse about what the purpose of support roles were. Roberts (1994) asked were 'they replacements for the nursing auxiliary, another form of enrolled nurse or actually a potentially cheaper version of the professionally qualified nurse?' (p. 24). As we have seen very little guidance was provided about support staff's scope of practice or educational requirements. Throughout the period how support workers were employed was left to the discretion of their employers. Given this, it is no surprise that there are recurring issues that characterise the NHS support workforce such as a lack of consistency in the tasks that they performed (Thornley, 1996). From the 1980s the NHS was subject to increased demand for its services as the population grew and aged, and generally shortages in staff. The lack of a coherent strategy towards the NHS's support workforce meant that the potential to use the role more strategically was not realised (Kessler et al., 2012). That strategy would finally be developed but only following a tragedy.

Robert Francis (2013) pointed out that a mini cab driver taking a patient to hospital or the security guard on the hospital door were subject to more regulation than NHS support workers. The issues raised by Francis (2013) had previously been identified by Fryer (2006) and were subsequently expanded on by Cavendish (2013) and reinforced by Willis (2015) just two years later. Despite the development of a national support workforce strategy in *Talent for Care*, it was the case that many support workers in 2015 were still facing the same issues their predecessors had. Of all the recommendations the four reviews made just two were taken forward – *The Care Certificate* and Nursing Associate (Skills for Health and Skills for Care did produce a code of practice and standards, although these had no force).

In 1994 Roberts referring to HCAs commented on the 'total absence of guidelines', including for entry-level requirements and the parameters of the role, creating a 'grey area' (p. 20). The period particularly from 2012 to 2015 was an opportunity to ensure that support staff were appropriately trained, deployed and developed in the NHS. That opportunity was missed.

Notes

1 Project lead June Mensah (February 2022), told me, 'The value of MSWs to maternity services is probably one of the most talk about topics, yet the career pathway for them is non-existent. We have a large amount of support workers across many specialities and yet their progression is so varied. They are often passed by in comment as "just the MSW"

but I want to say the maternity services would not do well without them. They work hard behind the varied coloured uniforms of the registered practitioners and also the very first person a service user may see, all of them set the scene for midwifery care within the National Health Services.'

2 Support staff employed in primary care are not covered by *Agenda for Change* – the national NHS pay and conditions agreement – and as we will see, are subject to a variety of pay arrangements.

3 See Box 5.6 for a description of the KSF.

References

Baker, D. (2019) Potential implications of degree apprenticeships for healthcare education, *Higher Education and Workplace Learning* 9(1), 2–17. https://doi.org/10.1108/HESWBL-01-2018-0006

Briggs, A. (1972) Report of the Committee on Nursing, Cmnd. 5115. London: HMSO.

Cavendish, C. (2013). *Cavendish Review. An Independent Enquiry into Healthcare Assistants and Support Workers in the NHS and Social Care Settings.* London: Department of Health. Available from: https://assets.publishing.service.gov.uk/government/uploads/system/uploads/attachment_data/file/236212/Cavendish_Review.pdf

Clark, I. (2014). Healthcare assistants, aspirations, frustrations and job satisfaction in the workplace. *Industrial Relations Journal* 45(4), 300–313.

Chartered Society of Physiotherapy (2014). *History of Support Workers within the CSP. Information Paper.* Available from: www.csp.org.uk/system/files/pd072_history_support_worker_within_csp.pdf

Daykin, N. and Clarke, B. (2000). 'They'll still get the bodily care'. Discourses of care and relationships between nurses and health care assistants in the NHS. *Sociology of Health & Illness* 22(3), 349 –363.

Department of Health (2000). *The NHS Plan: A Plan for Investment. A Plan for Reform.* London: HMSO. Available from: https://webarchive.nationalarchives.gov.uk/ukgwa/+/www.dh.gov.uk/en/publicationsandstatistics/publications/publicationspolicyandguidance/dh_4002960

Department of Health (2003). *Radiography Skills Mix. A Report on the Four-Tier Service Delivery Model.* London: Department of Health. Available from: https://webarchive.nationalarchives.gov.uk/ukgwa/+/www.dh.gov.uk/en/Publicationsandstatistics/Publications/PublicationsPolicyAndGuidance/DH_4007123

Department of Health (2004). *The National Services Framework Children, Young People and Maternity Services.* London: HMSO. Available from: www.gov.uk/government/publications/national-service-framework-children-young-people-and-maternity-services

Department of Health (2007). *Maternity Matters: Choice, Access and Continuity,* London: HMSO. Available from: https://dera.ioe.ac.uk/9429/7/dh_074199_Redacted.pdf

Department of Health (2010). *Widening participation into Pre-registration Nursing Programmes.* Available from: https://assets.publishing.service.gov.uk/government/uploads/system/uploads/attachment_data/file/213867/dh_116655.pdf

Edwards, M. (1997). The nursing aide: past and future necessity. *Journal of Advanced Nursing* 26, 237–245. DOI: 10.1046/j.1365-2648.1997.1997026237.x

Falconer, P. (2005). New Labour and the modernisation and public services. *Public Policy and Administration* 20(2), 81–85. https://doi.org/10.1177/095207670502000206

Ferlie, E., Ashburner, L., Fitzgerald, L. and Pettigrew, A. (1996). *The New Public Management in Action.* Oxford, Oxford University Press.

The Financial Times, 23 December 2021, available from: www.ft.com/content/43ba23b5-7dc3-435d-9d6a-201dbc038451

Ford, M. (2020). Government's 50,000 more nurses target 'insufficient for growing demand'. *Nursing Times,* 9 December 2021. Available from: www.nursingtimes.net/news/workforce/governments-50000-more-nurses-target-insufficient-for-growing-demand-09-12-2020/

Francis, R. (2013). Report of the Mid Staffordshire NHS Foundation Trust Public Inquiry. Available from: www.gov.uk/government/publications/report-of-the-mid-staffordshire-nhs-foundation-trust-public-inquiry

Fryer, R. (2006). *Learning for a Change.* London, Department of Health.

Griffin, R., Dunkley-Bent, J., Skewes, J. and Linay, D. (2010). Development of Maternity Support Worker Roles in the UK. *British Journal of Midwifery* 14 (4), 234–239. https://doi.org/10.12968/bjom.2010.18.4.47375

Griffin, R. (2018). Maximising the contribution of maternity support workers (MSWs) in North West London. *British Journal of Healthcare Assistants* 13(11), 549–551. https://doi.org/10.12968/bjha.2019.13.11.549

Griffin, R. (2021). *A Rewarding Job, but Frustrating Career. The Education, Development, and Deployment of Clinical Support Workers Employed in NHS Mental Health Services.* London: King's College London.

Halliday, K. Maskell, G. Beeley, L. and Quick, E. (2020). *Radiology. GIRFT Programme National Speciality Report.* Available from: www.gettingitrightfirsttime.co.uk/wp-content/uploads/2020/11/GIRFT-radiology-report.pdf

HEE. (2021). *Allied Health Professions' Support Worker Competency, Education, and Career Development Framework. Realising Potential to Deliver Confident, Capable Care for the future,* https://healtheducationengland.sharepoint.com/Comms/Digital/Shared%20Documents/For

Henshall, C., Doherty, A., and Green, H. (2018) The role of the assistant practitioner in the clinical setting: a focus group study. *BMC Health Serv Res* 18**,** 69, doi.org/10.1186/s12913-018-3506-y

Kessler, I. Heron, P. and Dopson, S. (2015). Professionalization and expertise in care work: The hoarding and discarding of tasks in nursing. *Human Resource Management,* 54(5), 737–752.

Kings College School of Nursing and Midwifery (2007). *Support Workers in Maternity Services: A National Scoping of NHS Trusts Providing Maternity Care in England.* London: Kings College London.

London South Bank University (2010). *The Impact of Maternity Care Support Workers in NHS Scotland.* NHS Education for Scotland.

HEE (2013). *Health Education England Mandate A Mandate from the Government to Health Education England (HEE) for April 2013 to March 2015.* Available from: www.gov.uk/government/publications/health-education-england-mandate

HEE (2014a). *Talent for Care. A National Strategic Framework to Develop the Healthcare Support Workforce.* Available from: www.hee.nhs.uk/sites/default/files/documents/TfC%20National%20Strategic%20Framework_0.pdf

HEE (2014b). *Widening Participation It Matters. Our Strategy and Initial Action Plan.* Available from: www.hee.nhs.uk/sites/default/files/documents/Widening%20Participation%20it%20Matters_0.pdf

HEE (2019). *Maternity Support Worker Competency, Education and Career Development Framework.* Available from: www.hee.nhs.uk/sites/default/files/document/MSW_Framework_MayUpdate.pdf

HEE. (2021a). *Allied Health Professions' Support Worker Competency, Education, and Career Development Framework. Realising Potential to Deliver Confident, Capable Care for the Future.* Available from: https://healtheducationengland.sharepoint.com/Comms/Digital/Shared%20Documents/Forms/AllItems.aspx?id=%2FComms%2FDigital%2FShared%20Documents%2Fhee%2Enhs%2Euk%20documents%2FWebsite%20files%2FAllied%20health%20professions%2FAHP%5FFramework%20Final%2Epdf&parent=

%2FComms%2FDigital%2FShared%20Documents%2Fhee%2Enhs%2Euk%20docume
nts%2FWebsite%20files%2FAllied%20health%20professions&p=true

HEE (2021b). *HEE Talent for Care*. [Website] Available from: www.hee.nhs.uk/our-work/tal
ent-care-widening-participation

HEE (n.d.). *What Comes Next? National Strategic Framework for Engagement with Schools and
Communities to Build a Diverse Healthcare Workforce*. Available from: www.hee.nhs.uk/
sites/default/files/documents/Strategic%20Framework%20-%20What%20Comes%20N
ext.pdf

Kantaris, X., Radcliffe, M., Acott, K., Hughes, P. and Chambers, M. (2020). Training
healthcare assistants working in adult acute inpatient wards in Psychological First Aid: An
implementation and evaluation study. *Journal of Psychiatric Mental Health Nursing 27*, 742–
751. DOI: 10.1111/jpm.12633

Kershaw, B. (1989). Project 2000. Identifying the nurse support worker. *Nursing Standard*
3(52), 40–43.

Kessler, I. and Heron, P., (2007). NHS modernisation and the role of HCAs. *British Journal
of Healthcare Assistants* 4(7), pp. 318–320, https://doi.org/10.12968/bjha.2010.4.7.48906

Kessler, I., Heron, P. and Dopson, S. (2012). *The Modernisation of the Nursing Workforce: Valuing
the Healthcare Assistant*. Oxford: Oxford University Press.

Kessler, I., Bach, S. and Nath, V. (2016). *Talent for Care: An evaluation*. London: King's College
London (unpublished).

Kessler, I. Heron, P. and Dopson, S., (2012). *The Modernisation of the Nursing Workforce: Valuing
the Healthcare Assistant*, Oxford: Oxford University Press.

Kessler, I., Heron, P. and Spilsbury, K. (2017). Human resource management innovation in
health care: the institutionalisation of new support roles. *Human Resource Management
Survey* 27(2), 228–245.

Kessler, I. and Spilsbury, K. (2019). The development of the new assistant practitioner role
in the English National Health Service: a critical realist perspective. *Sociology of Health &
Illness* 41(8), 1667–1684. https://doi.org/10.1111/1467-9566.12983

Kessler, I., Steils, N., Harris, J., Manthorpe, J. and Moriarty, J. (2021). *The Development of the
Nursing Associate Role: The Postholder Perspective*. NIHR Policy Research Unit in Health
and Social Care Workforce The Policy Institute, King's College London.

Kessler, I., Steils, N., Esser, A. and Grant, D. (2022). Understanding career development
and progression from a healthcare support worker perspective Part 2. *British Journal of
Healthcare Assistants* 16(1), 6–10. https://doi.org/10.12968/bjha.2022.16.1.6

Linay, D. and Lloyd, C. (2020). Shaping the NHS workforce. *British Journal of Healthcare
Assistants* 14(1), 20–23. https://doi.org/10.12968/bjha.2020.14.1.20

Meadows, S., Levenson, R. and Beaza, J. S. (2000). *The Last Straw: Explaining the NHS Nursing
Shortage*. London: Kings Fund. Available from: www.kingsfund.org.uk/sites/default/files/
laststraw.pdf

National Maternity Review (2016) *Better Births. Improving Outcomes of Maternity Services in
England. A Five Year Forward View for Maternity Care*. Available from: www.england.nhs.uk/
wp-content/uploads/2016/02/national-maternity-review-report.pdf

NHS Digital (2021). *NHS Workforce Statistics. April 2021*. Available from: https://digital.nhs.
uk/data-and-information/publications/statistical/nhs-workforce-statistics/april-2021.

NHS Education for Scotland (2020). *Healthcare Support Worker Learning Framework*. Available
from: www.nes.scot.nhs.uk/our-work/healthcare-support-workers-hcsws/

NHS Employers (n.d.). *National Profiles for Midwifery*. Available from: www.nhsemployers.
org/sites/default/files/2021-06/Midwifery-profile.pdf

NHS England. (2019). *The NHS Long Term Plan*. Available at: www.longtermplan.nhs.uk

NHS Modernisation Agency (2004). *10 High Impact Changes for Service Improvement and Delivery.* Available from: www.england.nhs.uk/improvement-hub/publication/10-high-impact-changes-for-service-improvement-and-delivery/

NHS Wales (2015). *Developing Excellence in Healthcare. An NHS Wales Skills and Competence Framework for Healthcare Support Workers in Nursing and the Allied Health Professions.* Available from: www.nwssp.wales.nhs.uk/sitesplus/documents/1178/HCSW%20Career%20Framework%20Nursing%20and%20Allied%20Health%20Professions.pdf

Nuffield Trust (2021a). *The NHS Workforce In Number* (Website). Available from: www.nuffieldtrust.org.uk/resource/the-nhs-workforce-in-numbers

Nuffield Trust (202ab). *Untapped? Understanding the Mental Health Clinical Support Workforce.* Nuffield Trust. Available from: www.nuffieldtrust.org.uk/research/untapped-understanding-the-mental-health-clinical-support

Nursing Times (2013). Minimum training standards for HCAs. Available from: https://cdn.ps.emap.com/wp-content/uploads/sites/3/2011/05/Francis-report-3.pdf

Rafferty, A. M. (1996). *The Politics of Nursing Knowledge.* London and New York: Routledge.

RCM (2011). *The Role and Responsibilities of MSWs.* RCM. Available from: www.rcm.org.uk/media/2338/role-responsibilities-maternity-support-workers.pdf

RCN (2007). The Regulation of Healthcare Support Workers. Available from: www.rcn.org.uk/about-us/our-influencing-work/policy-briefings/pol-1107

Richards, M. (2020). *Diagnostics: Recovery and Renewal.* Available from: www.england.nhs.uk/wp-content/uploads/2020/10/BM2025Pu-item-5-diagnostics-recovery-and-renewal.pdf

Roberts, I. L. (1994). The Health Care Assistant. Professional supporter or budget necessity? *Journal of Health Quality Assurance* 7(6), 20–25. DOI: 10.1108/09526869410059736

Skills for Health (2010). *Key Elements of the Career Framework.* Available from: https://skillsforhealth.org.uk/wp-content/uploads/2020/11/Career_framework_key_elements.pdf

Society and College of Radiographers (2002). *Scope of Practice of Assistant Practitioner.* Available from: www.sor.org/getmedia/4961def8-f45c-49a9-ae18-363ec8c4ccc6/Education%20and%20Professional%20Development%20Strategy_%20New%20Directions_1

Stewart-Lord, A., McLaren, S. M. and Ballinger, S. (2011). Assistant Practitioners' perceptions of the developing role and practice in radiography: Results from a national survey. *Radiography* 17, 193–200.

Stokes, J. and Warden, A. (2004). The changing role of the healthcare assistant. *Nursing Standard* 18(51), 33–37.

Thornley, C. (1996). *Poor Prospects. Local Pay Bargaining in Action.* London: Unison.

Thornley, C. (2007). Efficiency and equity considerations in the employment of Healthcare Assistants and support workers. *Social Policy and Society* 7(2), pp. 147–158.

United Kingdom Central Council for Nursing Midwifery and Health Visiting (1986). *Project 2000; a New Preparation for Practice.* United Kingdom Central Council for Nursing Midwifery and Health Visiting.

Wanless, D. (2002). *Securing Our Future Health: Taking a Long-Term View. Final Report.* Available from: www.yearofcare.co.uk/sites/default/files/images/Wanless.pdf

Willis, P. (2015). *Raising the Bar: Shape of Caring, A Review of the Future Education and Training of Registered Nurses and Care Assistants.* Available from: www.hee.nhs.uk/sites/default/files/documents/2348-Shape-of-caring-review-FINAL.pdf

WRES (2020). *Workforce Race Equality Standard. 2020 Data Analysis Report for NHS Trusts and Clinical Commissioning Groups.* Available from: www.england.nhs.uk/wp-content/uploads/2021/02/Workforce-Race-Equality-Standard-2020-report.pdf

2

MISSED OPPORTUNITIES?

The current position of NHS support workers

Introduction

The previous chapter set out a history of the NHS clinical support workforce up to the publication of the *Shape of Caring* review in 2015. This chapter brings the story up to date. As will be clear by now, whilst the research evidence about support workers is not extensive, what research there is, along with the formal reviews undertaken by Fryer (2006), Cavendish (2013) and Willis (2015), has revealed a consistent story of a workforce that is under invested in, often underappreciated and who face barriers to their progression. This continues. Commenting in 2021 The Health Foundation said that many

> lower paid NHS workers report a lack of opportunity to progress to better paid roles and say that they feel undervalued and unsupported at work, with a sense of feeling "invisible" unless something goes wrong. And while having a sense of autonomy at work is closely linked to job satisfaction, lower paid workers often feel they have no autonomy at all…Other factors affecting the health and wellbeing of lower paid staff include increased exposure to racial discrimination, being involved in physically demanding work or working with potentially hazardous materials such as in cleaning, laundry and catering roles.

Support workers employed in NHS mental health services described how they 'often feel undervalued and overlooked' and how they feel they 'deserve far more acknowledgment of their role and the value they bring to the NHS. Nurses are incredible, but [support workers] seem to get forgotten' (Griffin, 2021: 11).

Drawing on a number of academic disciplines, including labour market theory, this chapter will explore why the NHS clinical support workforce has and continues

DOI: 10.4324/9781003251620-4

to be 'forgotten'. The remaining chapters are concerned with what can be done to improve the situation.

What issues do support workers currently face?

In 2018 Griffin undertook a national survey, conducted semi-structured interviews, and organised focus groups to understand the experience of support workers employed in maternity services. MSWs reported that whilst on the one hand they derived considerable satisfaction form their work (in fact the word they most frequently used to describe their job was 'love'), there was no consistency or standardisation in how their roles were designed and deployed – even within organisations. There existed a plethora of job titles, a lack of consistent entry-requirements, poor access to occupationally relevant learning (just 6% of the survey respondents reported that they had accessed such learning), ill-defined role boundaries, along with a weak link between the tasks they performed and their grading. The majority of MSWs wanted to have greater development opportunities to contribute more to care.

MSWs in a focus group discussion expressed their frustrations: 'I absolutely love this job, but I think there is more that could be done to make us competent in our roles' and 'I love my role but sometimes I feel we're stuck' and 'My role has expanded over the years. My band is the same. I do love my job, but I find it hard to provide for my family on such a low income' (ibid., 14).

These frustrations were not restricted to support workers employed in maternity services. In 2020 the Health and Society Knowledge Exchange (HASKE) unit, based at the University of Cumbria, undertook a literature review in respect of AHP support staff, along with a series of deep dive interviews with employers who had purposively developed their support staff. Whilst HASKE found examples of good practice, alongside evidence of the positive impact of support staff made on organisational performance (see Box 2.1 below); they found that the AHP support workforce as a whole was characterised by a number of familiar issues, including a paucity of workforce data, lack of title, role and education requirement standardisation, an absence of workplace based routes into pre-registration healthcare degrees and a lack of organisational support, including funding, for training and protected time off to learn. Support worker scope of practice, the researchers wrote, was 'very much determined by the…service in which [support workers] are based and the specific needs of the patients in their care' (p. iii).

The Nuffield Trust (2021) found a similar story for support workers employed in mental health services, where they comprise around a third of that workforce, in a review of the published evidence and official data. Nuffield found that 96 separate titles existed for these support workers. This, they wrote, is 'potentially problematic, given titles can help indicate to both fellow workers and patients where responsibilities lie' (ibid., 14). A review by The Nuffield Trust of job adverts, and job descriptions found no consistency in the education and experience required in advertised posts. '[F]rom the mental health support worker job adverts we reviewed,' they wrote, 'qualifications listed as essential ranged from basic literacy and numeracy to a NVQ level 3 in a relevant subject.[1] While some variation might be reasonable given the different requirements of individual roles across specific settings, this warrants further investigation' they stated (ibid., 5). Other issues identified included inconsistent task allocation and poor access to education opportunities, once staff were employed. This matters they noted because support workers are likely to spend more time directly interacting with service users than any other member of staff. 'Lack of education, training and development opportunities contributes to poor quality care' (ibid., 8).

The issues identified by The Nuffield Trust (ibid.) echoed findings by other researchers of the mental health support workforce. Kantaris and colleagues (2020) reported that support workers could not access sufficient training and experienced limited supervision. Griffin (2021) through a national survey completed by over 370 support workers, identified a range of issues this workforce faced including that:

- Nearly a third of support workers surveyed wanted to progress their careers into higher support roles and almost a half into pre-registration degrees, but the majority did not know how to do so.
- Just 6% had started or completed an apprenticeship.
- A quarter had not had a development review with their manager in the last two years and only 36% of those that had had a discussion felt it was useful.

Perhaps as a consequence of these findings only 12% thought that the NHS valued the contribution of support workers.

Professor Sir Mike Richards' (2020) independent review of diagnostic radiography services found that, despite Assistant Practitioners being employed in the profession for nearly two decades, only 50% of services actually deployed the role. Even where services did deploy them, they did not do so in a consistent way, with support workers struggling to access education. Richards recommended an increase in the number of support workers employed in the profession.

Halliday and colleagues' (2020) deep dive review of radiography services found that even when Assistant Practitioners were employed there were a variety of approaches to their deployment resulting at times in unnecessary underutilisation. 'The responsibilities they [support workers] are given varies...This can mean that, at times, they are under-used, even when the rest of the team are extremely busy' (p. 37). As a result, 'few trusts benefit from the full opportunities [of support workers] to increase capacity' (p. 37). The study further found that support workers experienced a range of barriers to their development including lack of funding, along with

> a lack of clarity about how best to support training and in many cases the tension between releasing staff to participate in training and maintaining day-to-day workloads. While [employers] recognise the potential benefit of their people acquiring new skills, trusts may be unable to source adequate cover for their staff to allow them to attend the training course. This can even be an issue where funding has been secured.
>
> *p. 37*

In a similar vein, Stewart–Lord and colleagues (2018) questioned the extent to which the Assistant Practitioner role in radiography had been given the opportunity to fully realise its potential because of a lack of full integration and capacity to support its potential.

Turning to nursing, a review of the Nursing Associate role, which will be discussed in more detail in Chapter 7, found evidence of a lack of understanding of the role, inconsistency in its deployment and in the allocation of tasks, despite considerable national guidance on the role (Kessler et al., 2021).

The Health Foundation (2021) reviewed the results of the 2019 *NHS Staff Survey* and found that '52% of the overall [NHS] workforce felt involved in making decisions related to their area, team, or department, but only 39% of maintenance/ancillary staff and 41% of health care assistants felt the same way'. This research also pointed to the possible consequences of the barriers that support workers face, noting that the health and well-being of support staff are poorer than the workforce as a whole.

BOX 2.1 THE UTILISATION OF SUPPORT WORKERS IN PRIMARY CARE

The use of support workers in general practice became more widespread at the turn of the last century. In 2007 it was estimated that around a half of practices employed the role (Vail et al., 2011) with Bishop (2008) reporting that 6,000 support staff were employed in the sector in 2006. The expansion of support roles in primary care, mirrored a similar growth in Practice Nurses. Both roles were designed to relieve pressure on General Practitioners (Griffiths et al., 2010). A particular emphasis was placed on the role support staff could play in respect of health promotion and disease prevention targets (Vail et al., 2011).

Similar to the acute sector a decade earlier when the HCA role was first introduced following *Project 2000* (United Kingdom Central Council for Nursing Midwifery and Health Visiting, 1986), discussed in the last chapter, concerns were raised about role boundaries, threats to professional identity, cost-effectiveness, safety, delegation, competence and training as the role grew in number in primary care (Bosley and Dale, 2008). Concerns around role boundaries may have been compounded by the fact that the scope of practice for Practice Nurses was also unclear and shifting (Griffin et al., 2011).

An evaluation of a training programme designed for primary care support workers employed in general practice surgeries across East London found it led to a number of benefits. Following training support workers were able to expand the tasks that they could perform, and Practice Nurses were confident to delegate, thereby increasing capacity (Griffin et al., 2013). One support worker said of the programme: 'It is more flexible, more helping GPs, not to waste their time now with just taking blood pressure to diagnose hypertension and now I started seeing hypertension patients … We are taking bloods, taking blood pressure … we are advising healthy lifestyles.

Basically, the more we can do, we can take off them [nurses], so they can then take work off the GPs' (ibid., 461). Rather than blurring the boundaries with Practice Nurses, as had been feared (Bosley and Dale, 2008), the training allowed both support workers and Practice Nurses to more clearly understand each other's scope of practice – underlining the importance of occupationally relevant education to help codify role boundaries in the absence of national guidance. The support workers in the study also reported positive feedback from patients.

In a qualitative investigation, Vail and colleagues (2011) found that primary care support workers were generally positive about their work. Most had progressed into a patient facing role from a previous administrative one in their practice (an example of Grow Your Own workforce planning). Whilst enjoying their work, the support workers were dissatisfied about their pay levels, and felt that their role was not fully valued or utilised by the practice. They did, however, think that their role boundaries were clear and that they were positively received by patients. On pay a survey in practices based in south London found variations in hourly pay rates that ranged from £10.30/hour to £27.50/hour for general practice nurses and £6.72/hour to £13.00/hour for support workers (Ashwood et al.,, 2018). This study found that support workers were seen primarily as a supply route for future Practice Nurses.

Johnson and Moulton (2015) reported on a development programme in Stoke-On-Trent that was designed to develop the patient-facing support workforce in the area's 58 surgeries; deployment of which had up to that point been characterised by an inconsistency in the tasks undertaken by support workers between surgeries, due to variation in delegation. 'The blurring of defined roles within an ever-changing NHS has led to some nurse colleagues being uncertain as to what tasks their HCA colleagues can undertake as some of these are envisaged to be traditionally within the nursing domain. Giving practice nurses information on training content with a standardized approach will support delegation and teamwork', they reported (p. 304).

In 2019 general practices were reorganised into primary care networks (PCNs) each covering populations of between 30,000 and 50,000 people. PCNs work with other social care, community, mental health, hospital and voluntary services. In September 2021, a total of 137,119 (FTE) staff worked for general practice surgeries. Of these 16,183 were nurses and 6,657 support staff – almost 5% of the total primary care workforce, and 29% of the total nursing workforce (NHS Digital, 2021). It would appear that in the 20 years since clinical support roles were developed in primary care, their numbers have stalled, and they represent a smaller proportion of the workforce than in other NHS settings.

The evidence from recent research investigating the NHS clinical support workforce suggests that there has been little change in their experience of working in the NHS and as the Health Foundation (2021) and others (Griffin, 2021) point out the issues they face impact on their morale, sense of value and well-being; something we will return to in Chapter 6. This is not to say, of course, that there are not examples of good practice (HASKE, 2020), there are but these remain 'pockets of excellence' (Griffin, 2018: 46).

So far, the focus has been on issues and barriers. In the next section the positive impact that support staff can have on service delivery – if the issues we have been charting are addressed – will be considered.

What impact do support workers have on service outcomes?

The evidence for the impact of support workers on service outcomes is not extensive, reflecting a lack of studies rather than impact. In fact, investigations into the impact of this workforce only began to emerge in the early 2000s (NHS Confederation, 2011). However, what evidence there is shows the potential of the workforce to deliver a number of positive outcomes, including greater service capacity and quality of care. In a review of the literature undertaken in 2011 by Griffin and Sines, evidence has found that support workers employed in dementia care played a significant role in managing the environment on the ward, maintaining a more consistent emotional climate. Other research reported a link between the deployment of support staff and a reduced incidence of pressure ulcers, support workers employed on a nursing ward reduced the workload of nurses, improved teamworking and patient outcomes. In a review of the impact of Assistant Practitioners in 2011 the RCN reported their positive effect on service delivery, other staff, and performance. Spilsbury and colleagues (2011) also found that Assistant Practitioners improved the delivery of care.

Compared to other support roles, support workers in maternity services have been more extensively researched. These studies have identified the positive contribution MSWs can make to maternity care, including in public health, postnatal care, parent education, breast feeding support and assisting homebirths (for example London South Bank University, 2011; Kings Fund, 2011; and Griffin, 2020).

Griffiths and colleagues (2014) assessed peer reviewed studies investigating the link between nurses and support workers and patient outcomes for the National Institute for Health and Care Excellence (NICE) review of safe staffing evidence. They identified just eight studies, with mixed results. They did however find some evidence for the positive impact of support staff on reducing the risk of falls and incidence of pressure ulcers.

In radiography, although again the evidence is limited, reviews suggest that Assistant Practitioners have increased service capacity, freed up the time of, and enabled the development of, registered radiography roles (Stewart-Lord et al., 2011, and Palmer et al., 2015), as well as improving the continuity of care (Price et al., 2015). Halliday and colleagues (2020) found services 'using assistant practitioners to conduct image acquisition, releasing radiographer time to focus on reporting or on more complex modalities; training clinical support workers or imaging assistants to perform cannulation and help radiographers and radiology nurses prepare patients for a CT or MRI scan', with the benefit of minimising

> turnaround time between scanning and ensures there are no delays when the scanner is available; allowing trained clinical support workers or imaging assistants to vet patients for ultrasound, so that the sonographer doesn't have to. This then reduces the amount of time the sonographer has to dedicate to this 'administrative' task.

p. 36

HASKE (2020) interviewed a number of AHP services that had taken the strategic decision to actively develop their support workforce. Participants in the HASKE study reported that extending the scope of their support staff's practice increased capacity and freed up the time of registered staff to focus on 'more complex cases' (p. 50). This in turn enabled the running of more clinics, improved continuity of care, reduced waiting times and more physiotherapy sessions. Furthermore, deployment of support workers increased capacity for student placements. In terms of the quality of care, one participant in the HASKE (2020) study believed quality rose because – 'you are drawing on utilising the maximum potential of a really expert workforce' (p. 58). Finally, they found that investment in support staff reduced turnover and supported local GYO approaches which was seen as 'particularly beneficial for smaller [AHP] professions' which struggled to recruit (p. 50).

BOX 2.2 MAXIMISING THE CONTRIBUTION OF SUPPORT STAFF WORKING IN ORTHOPTIC SERVICES

HASKE (2020) found that services used Orthoptic Assistants for a range of tasks including setting up clinics, positioning equipment, liaising with patients, assess visual acuity and taking bloods. One 'of the main roles of the Orthoptic Assistant', one participant said, 'is to assess vision…that's taking a huge chunk of work away from orthoptists to allow us to do other assessments' (p. 53).

In primary care studies have identified a range of benefits associated with the employment of HCAs, including improved access to appointments, reduced waiting times, improvements in the quality of care for patients with long term conditions. increased capacity and patient satisfaction (Griffin et al., 2011; Vail et al., 2011; Griffin et al., 2013).

Support workers and safe staffing

One debate where the impact of support workers has been routinely considered is in discussions about safe staffing. Getting staffing levels and skill mix right across shifts is crucial to ensure patient safety and quality outcomes. NICE (2022) defines 'safe staffing' as occurring 'when reliable systems, processes and practices are in place to meet required care needs and protect people from missed care and avoidable harm'. Safe staffing centres on the following questions: How many staff should the NHS employ? What is the optimum staffing establishment for a department or team to ensure safety? What is the skill right mix between registered and support staff?

BOX 2.3 SKILL MIX

In healthcare skill mix can be understood as referring to (1) the different competences that staff possess, (2) as the ratio of one group of staff compared to another for example the proportion of General Practitioners and Practice Nurses employed, or nurses and support workers, or (3) the mix of staff within a service for example nurses and AHPs or midwives and nurses. 'Grade mix' refers to the proportion of different *Agenda for Change* pay bands within a service which may be a consequence of skill mix changes.

Skill mix changes occur through a number of mechanisms – through enhancing the responsibilities of an existing role within its existing scope of practice (for example a band 3 support worker who begins to take bloods), the substitution of one member of staff for another (replacing a nurse with a support worker or workers), the transferring of tasks from a more senior member of staff to a more junior one (for example a registered midwife no longer providing breast feeding support as the responsibility is delegated to a MSW) and finally, the creation of a completely new role, such as the Nursing Associate, which may undertake new tasks as well as tasks previously performed by others.

There are a number of decision-making tools available to assist NHS services to answer these questions, such the Mental *Health Optimal Staffing Tool* and the *Emergency Department Optimal Staffing Tool*. Two tools are NICE endorsed: *The Adult Inpatient Wards in Acute Hospitals* for nursing and *Birthrate Plus* for maternity (Box 2.5). Assuring patient safety is not, however, just a question of staff numbers, safety is also a consequence of developing a culture of safety, ensuring appropriate, reliable, and consistent processes and practices, and considering human factors in training. (Human factors are the things that can assist or inhibit effective and safe practice such as a lack of awareness or poor processes.)

BOX 2.4 SAFE STAFFING TOOLS

Developed in 2012 by The Shelford Group, the *Safer Nursing Care Tool* (SNCT) is based on services classifying patient acuity, including their risk of deterioration on a scale starting at Level 0 (patients whose needs are met by the provision of normal nursing care) to Level 3 (patients who need advanced care, respiratory support and/or therapeutic support). Against each classification a period of registered nursing time is allocated. Patients at Level 3 are judged to require five times the number of registered nursing time to support them than those at Level 0. These 'multipliers' include an uplift to take account of annual leave, sickness absence, supervision of students and so on. Services require sufficient staff in their establishment to ensure at any one-time factors such as annual leave are covered (The Shelford Group, n.d.).

The Shelford Group (n.d.) point out that no 'national workforce tool can incorporate all the factors' that determine how many staff should be deployed. For example, two similar wards with the same case mix are likely to require different establishments if one has more frequent admissions and ward attendees. Other factors to be considered include complaints, drug errors, infection rates and pressure ulcers, stressing the importance of professional judgement.

Founded on a peer-reviewed methodology, (for example Ball and Washbrook, 2010), Birthrate Plus is a framework for workforce planning and strategic decision-making that has been used by U.K. maternity units since 1988. Birthrate Plus. It has been described as the 'gold standard' (Yao et al., 2016) for maternity workforce planning, is NICE endorsed, and supported by the RCM and Royal College of Obstetrics and Gynaecology. Similar to the SNCT, Birthrate Plus assesses the acuity of women based on five categories and centred on a 1:1 ratio of women/registered midwives during birth. It takes account of factors influencing staff deployment including the geographical area covered by services, the need to supervise students and leave. Unusually the methodology does consider support workers and assumes that 10% of staffing complement can comprise other staff such as support workers.

Safe staffing decision tools, such as those described in Box 2.5, primarily focus on the numbers of registered staff needed. Is there, though, a link between the proportion of support workers employed compared to registered staff (skill mix), and patient outcomes? A number of studies (in nursing) have suggested that there could be a negative association between the support worker staffing numbers and patient outcomes (see Robb et al., 2011).

Griffiths and colleagues (2014) in their review of the evidence on the link between nursing staffing levels and patient safety, identified eight studies directly addressing this question. The results were mixed. Three studies found no link between the number of nursing support workers employed compared to registered nurses and (1) mortality, (2) failure to rescue or (3) falls. Four studies did, though, find an association between staffing levels and rates of fall. Finally, of three studies reviewing the impact of skill mix on pressure ulcers, one found an incidence of higher levels when there were more support workers employers, another found levels were lower and a third found no link.

Reviewing the safe staffing literature, Griffin and Sines (2012) noted limitations in the methodology deployed by such studies, including a failure to take account of different patient needs or unobserved variables. It is impossible to know often from the data used, for example, whether poor patient outcomes are due to too few nurses and too many support workers or too few support workers *and* too few nurses or just too few nurses (ibid.). Clearly any member of staff – registered or not – whose workload is too high may have their ability to observe patients impaired.

Where service outcomes do appear to be negatively impacted on by skill mix, the issue may not be one of capacity (numbers) but rather capability (knowledge and skills). As we have repeatedly seen support workers have variable and inconsistent access to education and this can have an impact on the quality of care (Nuffield Trust, 2021). It would be reasonable to assume that a support worker who has been appropriately trained to, for example, prevent falls within a well-designed and supported job, and who is also appropriately supervised and delegated tasks too, will be able to contribute more to reducing fall rates than one who has not been trained. Safe staffing studies have not been able to gather detailed data on support workers such as their banding and training, tending to conflate all roles together. An untrained member of staff employed at band 2, will not have the same capability to, for example, observe deterioration in a patient on a ward as a band 3 with an occupationally relevant qualification and Continuing Professional Development (CPD). These points were made by Edwards, as long ago as 1997, who pointed out that many skill mix studies compared trained nurses with untrained support staff raising 'doubts about the validity of those…studies that attempt to compare the quality and effectiveness of qualified versus unqualified nurses' (p. 241).

None of this, of course, is to say that there should not be sufficient numbers of registered staff in settings, but rather to suggest that the issue of skill mix, and safety is complex and requires further detailed research in the context of support worker role design and deployment.

NHS workforce planning

Effective workforce planning means ensuring 'the right people, with the right competences are in the right jobs at the right time' to meet the current and future demand for services (Willis et al., 2018: 250). Demand for NHS services continues to rise as the population grows, life expectancy lengthens, and medical advances mean that a wider range of treatments are available. Whilst people are living longer, they are not necessarily living well, with many suffering from long-term and chronic conditions such as obesity and heart disease (Prime Minister's Office and Department of Health and Social Care, 2022).

Workforce planning matters in all organisations, but perhaps particularly so in the NHS (and social care) because healthcare delivery is 'people and skills-intensive' (Charlesworth and Lafond, 2017: 2). Failure to get workforce planning right threatens the NHS's delivery of care over the next decade (NHS England, 2019a – see p. 29).

Getting workforce planning 'right', though, has long been a challenge for the NHS – as first noted by the Briggs Committee in 1972. Half a century and more after it remains a, perhaps, the challenge the NHS faces (see Addicott et al., 2015, and Buchan et al., 2019, for contemporary discussions of the shortcomings of NHS workforce planning processes and their consequences). An ex-Secretary of State for Health went as far as to call NHS workforce planning a 'joke' (O'Dowd, 2021). The House of Commons Health Select Committee that Jeremy Hunt made that comment too, called NHS workforce planning 'opaque' and pointed out that there remained a lack of clear targets across specialisms for how many staff the NHS will be required in the future.

The NHS Long Term Plan (NHS England, 2019a) acknowledged that workforce planning processes have been 'disjointed' and that 'over the past decade, workforce growth has not kept up with need, and the way staff have been supported to work has not kept up with the changing requirements of patients' (p. 78). One consequence of this is that the NHS has had to rely on international recruitment to fill the gap. In 2020 15% of NHS staff were non-UK residents (Rolewicz and Palmer, 2021). Even so, workforce capacity has not kept up with demand (ibid.).

The *NHS Interim People Plan* (NHS England, 2019b) set out the challenge that workforce planning poses in healthcare, noting that even

> medium-term workforce planning [can] be challenging for a system as large and complex as the NHS. It is intrinsically difficult to predict future NHS funding, patient needs, potential scientific and technological advances, and changes in service models over the time horizon that it takes to train clinical professional.
>
> *p. 47*

The 'failures' (Buchan, 2007: 7) and 'problems' (Charlesworth and Lafond, 2017: 3) associated with NHS workforce planning derive, in part, from the service's complex and multifaceted nature: the large number of services provided, their configurations and multiple care pathways, system delays (such as the time lag in training staff like nurses), along with the challenge of forecasting future demand (Willis et al., 2018). Additionally, there is a need to balance service-led demand with available financial resources in the public sector (Buchan, 2007).

From this book's perspective a further point needs to be made. NHS workforce planning has overwhelmingly focused on what one article on the subject described as the 'skilled' and 'highly regulated' workforce (Charlesworth and Lafond, 2017: 3). *The NHS Interim People Plan* (NHS England, 2019b) when discussing workforce planning referred to 'clinical professionals' and, as we will see, contained very few references to support staff. Support worker roles, with the exception, to some extent, of Assistant Practitioners and more recently Nursing Associates, have largely been excluded from the policy and processes associated with NHS workforce planning (The Nuffield Trust, 2021). Given the failures of workforce planning in the NHS more generally, this has without doubt compounded the problems support workers can face.

BOX 2.5 KLUDGES – AN EXPLANATION FOR THE FAILURES OF NHS WORKFORCE PLANNING?

The Oxford English Dictionary defines a kludge as a collection of poorly-matching parts, and, 'a machine, system, or program that has been improvised or "bodged" together; a hastily improvised and poorly thought-out solution to a fault or "bug"'. As this definition implies the term is frequently used in computing. Steven Teles (2013) applied the concept to public policy in liberal democracies, where he argued, successive governments, rather than address policy issues afresh tend to 'bolt on' a new assemblage to existing policy, further denting the policy's original purpose.

This concept, in my view, sheds light on problems with workforce planning in the NHS. Consider the agencies that have existed with responsibility for NHS workforce supply (and education commissioning) between 2000 and 2020. The list begins with Workforce Development Confederations which, in 2002, were merged with Strategic Health Authorities (SHAs) who were responsible for service planning. Whilst SHAs continued until 2013, their numbers were reduced (in London from five to one, for example). SHA's workforce responsibilities were then taken over by HEE, which originally had a regional focus (with five offices, called Local Education and Training Boards, in London, for instance) but was then subject to two major reorganisations in its short life (creating, firstly, two offices in London and then one). In 2022 HEE was subsumed into NHS England. This is not the full story, however. In 2020 there were also Regional People Boards (run by HEE and NHS England) and Integrated Care System (ICS) People Boards (previously Local Workforce Advisory Boards) also concerned with workforce along with a number of national initiatives. It is perhaps not a surprise that the *Health and Care Act* (2021) placed a responsibility on the Secretary of State to publish a report describing the system in place for assessing and meeting the workforce needs of the NHS.

It is not just operating models that are subject to kludges – individual policy can be fragmented, ill-assorted and, frankly, 'bodged' together. Consider the introduction of the regulated Nursing Associate role. Whilst broadly recommended by Willis (2015) the actual role created by HEE was different to the one he recommended. The recommendation to create the role did not exist in isolation to other recommendations he made in respect of support staff, like the need for transferable learning and consistent role boundaries. All of these though were ignored. Perhaps most significantly the relationship between Nursing Associates and Assistant Practitioners was not clarified.

Failure to get workforce planning processes right has negative implications for service delivery, resource allocation, existing staff and safety (Lopes et al., 2015). The impact on existing staff was graphically illustrated during Covid-19, when poor workforce planning led staff shortages was attributed as a major factor contributing to staff burnout by a House of Common Select Committee in 2021 review: '[a]t the heart of the solution to workforce burnout and resilience is one simple change, without which the situation is unlikely to improve: the need for better workforce planning'.

The most recent workforce planning iteration in the NHS was trailed in 2019, when *The NHS Interim People Plan* (NHS England, 2019b) was published setting out how the workforce implications of *The NHS Long Term Plan* (NHS England, 2019a), published earlier that year, would be met. A new workforce planning operating system emerged with planning more focused on local systems, complemented by national strategies, such as international recruitment and return to practice.

The details of this workforce planning system will be discussed in detail shortly. Whether it delivers the staffing the healthcare service needs remains to be seen, however there is no question that the increased role of ICS, is a significant change for support worker recruitment and development. As we have seen (Chapter 1) many support workers are recruited from local labour markets and as will see (Chapter 3) local employment and skills partners, such as local authorities, have a significant role to play in recruiting and up-skilling support workers.

Current NHS workforce policy: The NHS Long Term Plan, People Plans and The Health and Care Act

The NHS Long Term Plan published by NHS England in January 2019 signalled the start a series of reforms culminating in the 2022 *The NHS Health and Care Act*, that have substantially reshaped the way the NHS is organised, including its approach to workforce planning. The most significant overall change was a move away from a commissioning system based on competition between service providers (first introduced by the *Health and Care Act* in 2012 – the so-called 'Lansley reforms' named after the then Health Secretary) to one based on collaboration. The Act sought to join health and social care services closer together and refocus planning on *improving* health rather than just *providing* health services. It also increased the powers of the Secretary of State, including in respect of local service reconfiguration as well as putting ICSs on an official legal footing.

Surprisingly given the staffing issues faced by the NHS, the Act contained very few references to workforce, something the Kings Fund (2021) described as a 'weakness' when it was published. It did, however, provide an obligation on the Secretary of State to describe the system for assessing and meeting the workforce needs, although this obligation fell short of a requirement to state how many staff are needed to meet demand. The most significant change for workforce, particularly support workers, resulted indirectly from the enhanced role of ICSs. This was spelt out in *The 2021/22 NHS Operating Plan* (NHS England, 2021) which called on ICS's to 'develop and deliver local workforce supply plans with a focus on both recruitment and retention, demonstrating effective collaboration between employers to increase overall supply, widen labour participation in the health and care system and support economic recovery' (p. 5). How this aspiration might be met is the subject of Chapter 3.

BOX 2.6 WHAT ARE INTEGRATED CARE SYSTEMS?

ICSs are partnerships between organisations concerned with the health and care needs of a local population. Partners, including the NHS, local authorities and the voluntary, community and social enterprise sector, work together to plan and deliver interventions aimed at reducing health inequalities and addressing population health needs. Although in existence in various forms since 2018, ICSs were only put on a formal legal setting in 2022. Like SHAs before them, ICSs bring together service and workforce needs locally (see Chapter 3 for a discussion of the implications of this for recruitment into the NHS and the role of the NHS as an 'anchor institution').

The key governing bodies of ICSs are the Integrated Care Board (ICB) and Integrated Care Partnership (ICP). ICP members include public health, housing services and the voluntary sector. They are responsible for developing a joined-up strategy setting out how the care needs of the local population will be met. ICSs also have a People Board concerned with ensuring that local providers have enough staff with the right skills to deliver the strategy through an ICS workforce plan. *The NHS Interim People Plan* (NHS England, 2019b) set out a 'vision for people who work for the NHS to enable them to deliver the *NHS Long Term Plan*' (p. 2). The workforce role of ICSs, working with partners, was defined as in that document as:

1. Developing long term population-based workforce plans.
2. Supporting the delivery of national education policies such the training of doctors and placement infrastructure.
3. Providing leadership.
4. Coordinating action to reduce reliance on temporary staffing.
5. Delivering initiatives locally to make the NHS a better place to work.
6. Improving staff recruitment and retention.
7. Working closely with local authorities, social care and public health agencies on shared workforce priorities.
8. Overseeing the development of primary care networks.
9. Maintaining and improving social partnership working with trade unions locally.

In addition to setting out the new workforce planning operating model (see Box 2.7) *The NHS Interim People Plan* (NHS England, 2019b) set out the human resource issues the NHS needed to address. These included 'rising levels of bullying and harassment', the poor experiences of BAME NHS staff, high sickness absence rates and staff frustration at not having enough time to treat patients (p. 4). *The NHS Interim People Plan* (ibid.) also set out a series of specific workforce needs and targets.

What it did not do, to any large extent, was to specifically address the needs of the NHS support workforce. Beyond a pledge to increase the number of Nursing Associates and the use of apprenticeships, (which are available to all NHS staff), the 40% of the NHS support workforce employed in clinical roles hardly got a look in. This was also the case with the *NHS Long Term Plan* (NHS England, 2019a) whose chapter on workforce barely mentioned support staff, beyond a pledge to increase apprenticeships 'with an expectation that employers will offer all entry-level jobs as apprenticeships before considering other recruitment options' (p. 81).

To be fair other workforce developments flagged in both documents did have implications for support workers including, as we have discussed, the enhanced role of ICSs in workforce planning and the call for the NHS to 'use its role as an anchor institution to create employment opportunities in local communities for school leavers, those will disabilities and those looking to switch career' (p. 50), but the support workforce, not for the first time, remained conspicuous by its absence in the both key policy documents.

It may have been that the workforce implementation plan promised for 2019 (NHS England, 2019a) which was due to follow *The NHS Interim People Plan* (NHS England, 2019b), would have more explicitly addressed support worker development. It was proposed that this plan, supported by a national workforce group, would consider the whole NHS workforce, as well as the needs of individual groups. However, the Covid-19 pandemic meant that although work on the plan had begun, it was not published. Instead in 2020, NHS England published *Our People Promise* which set out a series of pledges the NHS should meet by 2024. Whether the NHS has met these will be judged by the results of the NHS Staff Survey. *Our People Promise* committed the NHS to be:

1.   A compassionate and inclusive place to work, for example where any form of discrimination, bullying or violence is not tolerated.
2.   A workplace where staff are recognised and rewarded for what they do.
3.   A workplace that staff will feel able to speak up.
4.   A safe and healthy place to work.
5.   A workplace where staff shall have 'plentiful' and equal opportunities to learn and develop and the NHS attracts people to work for it from a range of diverse backgrounds.
6.   A workplace where staff are supported to work flexibly.
7.   A workplace where people work together as a team.

These goals are not only laudable, but also address key issues that support workers can face, including unequal access to learning, a lack of voice and not being fully integrated into teams. Again, though, it remains to be seen how these pledges are translated into tangible changes, particularly given the on-going NHS workforce crisis and lack of linked policy to deliver all these objectives.

On 22 November 2022, it was announced by the Department of Health and Social Care that HEE would be merged into NHS England, along with the NHS's digital agency NHSX – in order to put 'workforce and technology at the heart of long-term planning' (Neville, 2021). HEE was first established as a SHA in June 2012 and became a Non-Departmental Public Body of the Department of Health and Social Care in 2015. It was responsible for planning, training, and developing the existing and future NHS workforce through the work of its national and regional teams.

UK employment and skills policy

So far, we have considered the NHS support workforce from the perspective of healthcare policy and history alone. That is not, however, the whole story. In terms of employment and skills, the NHS does not exist in isolation, (although as the UK's largest employer it can feel sometimes like it does). Developments in what is known as vocational education and training (see Box 2.7 below) and employment more generally affect support workers. Indeed, 'some of the barriers to effective learning support workers face, such as the need for greater flexibility in the delivery of apprenticeships or increased investment in further education, need to be resolved via wider policy reform' (Kessler et al., 2020: 10). The next chapter will discuss in some detail the benefits for the NHS in working more closely with the Further Education (FE) sector particularly in respect of employment, this section will briefly describe recent reforms to FE, which ICSs should be well placed to engage with. This section will briefly discuss recent developments in the skill system.

BOX 2.7 WHAT IS VOCATIONAL EDUCATION AND TRAINING (VET)?

VET refers to any formal learning whose objective is to provide people with the knowledge, skills and behaviours they need to either perform a job they are employed in, or to progress their careers, retrain, or, if unemployed or economically inactive, to gain employment. Examples of VET programmes include Technical Levels, Business and Technology Education Council (BTEC) qualifications and apprenticeships. The case could be made that much healthcare-related learning is VET; healthcare degrees, after all, include a significant 'hands-on' practical element through placements; however, VET normally refers to learning up to and including RQF level 5.

In July 2021 the prime minister Boris Johnson promised, as part of his government's 'levelling up' agenda, 'to escalate the value of practical and vocational education'

(Staton et al., 2021). In the foreword to the 2021 White Paper, *Skills for Jobs*, the then Secretary of State for Education stated, 'this country has not always shown further education the esteem it deserves, with too many people – and too many employers – wrongly believing that studying for a degree at university is the only worthwhile marker for success' (Department of Education, 2021: 3).

Concerns about the quality of vocational education, which is largely delivered by the FE sector, are nothing new. An 1880s Royal Commission unfavourably contrasted the standard of education among 'workmen' in England with that in Germany (Staton et al., 2021). Recently FE has experienced a prolonged period of under investment, including a 50% cut in spending between 2010 and 2021. The total annual £3.5 billion budget for FE in 2021 was less than Oxford and Cambridge universities combined (IFS, 2021). Partly as a result of reduced funding, the numbers of people studying in the FE sector fell from just under 4 million in 2005/06 to below 2 million in 2020 (Hubble et al., 2021).

BOX 2.8 COLLEGES

In 2020 one million adults and 652,000 young people aged 16–18 study in college, studying a wide range of subjects at different academic levels:

- 34% study a RQF level 2 or below qualification.
- 33% a RQF level 2 qualification.
- 23% a RQF level 3 qualification.
- 10% a qualification at RQF level 4 or above (including degrees).

There were 350,000 students studying a health care qualification in colleges in 2020. Whilst the majority of people in FE study or train in colleges, the sector includes other providers such as local authorities, independent training providers and employers.

Source: NHS Confederation and College of
The Future (2020) and Hubble et al. (2021)

The problems experienced in FE were compounded by poor estates and low salary levels. FE lecturers earned an average £13,000 less a year than their colleagues in HE (Augar, 2019). The sector has also been subject to considerable policy volatility (ibid.). Writing in 2017, Norris and Adam noted that since 1980 FE had been subject to 28 major pieces of legislation and been led by 48 Secretary of States – totals that have both risen in the subsequent years (another example of a 'kludge' approach to public policy).

In October 2021, the *Skills and Post-16 Education Bill* was introduced into Parliament. In addition to the employer-centred proposals trailed in the *Skills for*

Jobs White Paper the Bill set out that the majority of technical qualifications would be designed by employers by 2030. The Bill also set out:

- Proposals to support lifelong learning through the provision, from 2025, of flexible loans to support retraining.
- Measures to allow the government to intervene if providers are judged to be delivering poor outcomes.
- Boosting recruitment into FE and professional development for existing staff.

Chapter 3 will discuss in depth the opportunities the NHS can benefit from engaging with local employment and skill systems and their institutions such as colleges. The reforms to VET should assist this.

Making sense of the development of the NHS support workforce

It is now time to take stock. The history of the NHS support workforce is one of enduring issues, such as poor job design and limited access to education. These issues – and their solutions were clearly articulated in the reviews undertaken by Fryer (2006), Cavendish (2013) and Willis (2015). These issues, though, continue and anyone wishing to enhance the contribution of support staff will, more likely than not, need to address them whether nationally, across an ICS or on a hospital ward or in a general practice surgery. In academic terms the deployment of support staff can be said to be 'path dependent', meaning that it is the result of decisions, events and policy (or perhaps more importantly a lack of policy) made in the past. Very little of the history of support staff has been driven by the needs of the workforce itself and the contribution it can make to patient care, but rather by external factors particularly staffing shortages and moves to close the professions. As a consequence, support staff have frequently been seen in a subordinate position as 'aides', 'helpers' and 'assistants' – even though they often provide the bulk of face-to-face care.

The remaining section of the chapter will consider why the support workforce has been treated in the way that it has, what the significance and consequence of that may be and how it can be approached by those seeking to enhance the contribution of support workers.

A simple answer to the question – why have support workers been treated the way they have – is poor workforce planning and the fact that their recruitment, the tasks they perform, their grading, titles and career development opportunities have been determined by local employers. As we have seen workforce planning in the NHS has flaws and has tended to ignore support workers. This has resulted in a fragmented and inconsistent approach to this workforce, most graphically illustrated by the plethora of titles that exist, but also by the lack of transferability of learning and inconsistent job design. No doubt the wider weaknesses inherent within the UK vocational education and training system has played its part. These explanations, though, do not adequately go to the heart of the matter. Why have successive governments largely left the development of a significant part of the NHS's workforce to local employers? Why do national workforce planning and strategies so often exclude support workers?

A meta problem

Before we consider possible answer, it needs to be stated that the issues support workers face are complex. By that I mean they *multi-faceted, multi-agency* and *interrelated*. HASKE (2020) described the support worker landscape as 'varied and complex' (p. i). The issues we have considered have built up over a long period of time. However, whilst they are complex, they do not represent a 'wicked problem'. Wicked problems can be defined problems that have multiple causes, are hard to define and lack a clear, or in some cases any, answer (Camillus, 2008). This does not describe the problems support workers face. In contrast support worker issues are very well defined. The repetition of the issues they face revealed in research and reviews, frankly borders on the tedious. Nor are these issues novel. Quite the opposite. Plenty of private and public sector organisations employee staff at the same education levels as NHS support workers yet manage to appropriately develop them. Moreover, the issues support workers face are structured. They are, in my view, best defined collectively, not as a wicked problem, but rather as a 'meta-problem' – a problem of problems (Dror, 1971). A series of problems conflate to restrict the contribution support staff make to care. For example, if support worker jobs are poorly defined, then their scope of practice will not be clear or consistent. This will impact on registered staff's decisions to delegate tasks. The problem may be further compounded by either an absence or unawareness of relevant educational programmes, limiting the value of development reviews staff have with their managers and so on. The individual problems combine to create a meta-problem. Think of a ball of string that is tangled up and needs unwinding.

A feature of meta-problems is that addressing one individual problem alone will only have a partial impact on the overall problem. Pulling one thread free of the tangled ball of string will not unwind it all. So, for example even if every single support worker in the NHS completed *The Care Certificate* (which they have not) or accessed an apprenticeship (which is also not the case), this would not address all the range of issues this workforce faces. This is why such policy interventions that have taken place addressed at support workers have had limited impact. They do not address all the threads. Meta-problems also require time to resolve simply because collectively they can be too big to tackle in one go (Dror, 1971).

Understanding support worker development as a meta problem can assist strategies to enhance their contribution. Box 2.9 below sets out some methods that can be used to address complex and meta issues.

BOX 2.9 HOW TO TACKLE A COMPLEX META PROBLEM LIKE SUPPORT WORKER DEVELOPMENT

There are a number of tools that can assist the tackling of meta problems, such as design thinking (the following draws extensively from Kelley and Kelley, 2013). Design thinking can be defined as a methodology for practical, creative resolution of problems or issues that look for an improved future result, in this case building support worker capacity and capability. At the heart of the idea is *empathy*. Design thinking begins with a project's outcome and seeks to redefine this as a 'challenge' question, empathetic to end users. Rather than asking, for example: 'how do we improve support worker training?', the question could be reframed from the perspective of the end user and posed instead as 'how can we ensure the local population receive safe, effective, compassionate and high-quality care from support workers?' Kelley and Kelley (ibid.) suggest projects based on design thinking adopt the following steps:

1. Create a shared understanding of the issue that needs to be resolved and what success comprises.
2. Review the problem through research or talking to stakeholders.
3. Generate as many ideas (called 'ideation') as possible to solve the problem discarding none at this stage.
4. Identify ideas from stage 3 that could be tested.
5. Review and then choose the idea(s) to implement remembering that the apparently most practical solutions are not always the best.
6. Implement the idea(s).
7. Evaluate to determine if the idea(s) meet the goal(s) agreed step 1, learning from feedback and data collected.

Drawing on design thinking but with fewer steps Discovery Methodology is another useful approach anyone concerned with support worker development might adopt when seeking to improve their capacity and capability. Discovery involves three steps:

Step 1 – Set a goal

This might be 'recruiting more local people into entry-level roles' or 'increase capacity and capability' or 'widening access to pre-registration'. Where partners are involved in the project ensure there is a consensus on the goal.

Step 2 – Define the problem(s)

What is stopping the goal from being achieved? Constraints need to be considered from various perspectives, including support workers, their managers, education providers and service users. Widening access to pre-registration degrees, for example, may appear a very different issue from the perspective of a university receiving many applications from A Level students for their course, compared to a support worker wishing to progress her career. Defining the problem(s) allows the context enabling or inhibiting the meeting of the goal to be understood, as well as helping to drive solutions, the next stage.

Step 3 – Solutions

In identifying the need to build capacity to meet rising demand for diagnostic radiography services, Richards (2020) argued that a 'blank sheet' approach needed to be taken to workforce planning in radiography. Given the path dependent nature of the support workforce this makes sense and applies to the last stage of Discovery Methodology. Solutions need to be found to address the constraints identified in Step 2 and achieve the goal, but this may require fresh thinking.

Turning now to the deeper question of why the NHS support workforce has developed in the way that it has creating a meta-problem, there is, as far as I am aware, no research directly investigating this question. The remainder of this chapter draws on labour market, sociology and learning theory for insights. We will consider whether support workers represent a secondary labour market in the NHS, whether they can be perceived in terms of institutional approaches to the acceptance or rejection of new roles and finally consider what Fuller and Unwin's (2003 and 2011) conceptualisation of workplace restrictive or expansive learning cultures can tell us about the treatment of support staff.

Is the NHS a segmented labour market?

Skill systems are characterised by decisions about the division of labour made by the state, firms, associations and education providers (Busemeyer and Trampush, 2011). These decisions can lead to variable outcomes in different parts of the labour market, so that skills formation in the NHS for a doctor may be different to that for a nurse and both different to that for a support worker. This points to the potential of a segmented labour market existing. Segmentation means that different parts of a labour market are treated differently with features such as pay, allocation of work, progression opportunities, employment rights and status determined by institutional and social factors rather than, as neoclassical economics suggests, the value of human capital itself. In other words, support workers are treated in accordance with societal assumptions about the status of their work and, indeed, themselves, rather than the contribution of their labour itself, which as Cavendish (2013) said, is frequently fundamental to care.

Segmentation can occur across the whole economy, within or between sectors and industries and within organisations. Segmented labour markets comprise a primary (core) segment and a secondary (periphery) segment. It is suggestive that the NHS clinical workforce is described in a dualistic way, as we have discussed, for example as 'registered' and 'unregistered' staff or the 'regulated' and 'unregulated'

TABLE 2.1 Features of segmented labour markets and the NHS

Primary (Registered)	Secondary (Unregistered)
Regulated	Unregulated
Recruited nationally from Higher Education	Recruited locally
National progression routes	Local progression routes
National sanctioned qualifications	Employer determined qualifications
Access to in-work training (CPD)	Poor access to in-work training
High status/value	Low status/low value
Female dominated	Female dominated
Ethnically diverse	Ethnically diverse

or as 'trained' and 'untrained'. Moreover, the very notion of a 'support' role, as conceived in the NHS, is of a role that is subordinate, secondary or even inferior to registered ones.

As Table 2.1 above shows a case can indeed be made that the NHS clinical workforce is in fact segmented, at least in part, with support workers located in a secondary market displaying many of the classic characteristics of such markets, one feature of which is that it is difficult to transition from one segment to the other (Turnbin et al., 2014). This is certainly an issue for NHS support staff (see Willis, 2015 for example) who struggle to progress into pre-registration degrees – the entry point for the primary market. Different segments are treated differently, with the primary one more privileged that the secondary. An example of differentiated treatment was when, in 2019, the NHS received a £150 million increase in funding for CPD, but the funding was only made available to registered staff (Kessler et al., 2020).

Segmented labour markets tend to be based on class, gender or ethnicity, or frequently interrelated differences (Bradley, 2015). Is this the case in the NHS?

In respect of gender 'men and women work in different jobs, and often do so in different organisations' (Jacobs, 1999: 125), with so-called 'women's work' being lower paid and of a lower status than men's (Bradley, 2015). Thornley (2007), amongst others, has noted that the nursing support workforce is female dominated with 'the usual implications for the undervaluation of "women's work"' (p. 150). Taking the NHS as a whole and comparing the sector with the wider labour market, the gendering of employment around 'emotional work,' which is often associated with 'body work' (ibid.), would seem to play a part in shaping comparative pay levels, and prospects but for *both* registered and unregistered staff alike. Both the registered and unregistered clinical workforces are female dominated.

If gender does not appear to explain the existence of a segmented labour market in the NHS, does ethnicity? Again, it does not appear that the unregistered workforce is any more or less diverse than the registered one, with 18.3% of band 2 staff being from BAME backgrounds and 15.5% of band 3s, compared to 27.5% of band 5s, 18% of band 6s and 15% of band 7s (WRES, 2020).

The differences between the primary and secondary labour markets in the NHS, may be a result of the socio-economic backgrounds of staff in each segment, rather than race or gender. Whilst data on the class characteristic of this workforce does not exist, the NHS support workforce does appear to display elements of the class-based characteristics of segmented labour markets more generally (Eidlin, 2015). For example, whilst support workers have always been able to join trade unions such as Unison, they were not until recently allowed to be members of professional bodies. The fact that support workers are more likely to be recruited from local labour markets, and join NHS employment directly from school or college rather than university or after working in another sector particularly retail and hospitality (Kessler and Heron, 2007 and Kessler et al., 2021) is suggestive of the (working) class-origin of this workforce, and in part may explain the way that the workforce has been treated, compared to registered staff.

Whilst the concept of a segmented labour market does appear a helpful way to understand the position of support workers and their treatment and, as Table 2.1 shows, the NHS clinical workforce as a whole does display many of the characteristics of a segmented labour market, it does differ from traditional understandings of labour segmentation in some ways.

The concept of 'imagined futures' refers to the capacity of an individual 'to look forward and envisage possibilities for themselves' (Kessler et al., 2016: 4). The extent to which this happens can drive individual behaviours in the workplace (such as seeking learning opportunities) as well as social identity. Characteristically, workers in secondary labour markets do not have high expectations of what they think they can achieve in their careers. Kessler, Nath and Bach's (ibid.) research suggest this is not the case for NHS support workers. Working in such close proximity to registered staff, support workers *can* imagine and aspire to a future where they become a registered healthcare professional. As Chapter 7 will show many support workers hold that aspiration, however they are realistic about the actual chances of them achieving this.

Whether there is a fully segmented labour market in the NHS is perhaps debatable. 'The labour market within the healthcare sector is complex… [at lower levels] there remain aspects of an almost secondary market with low status and limited training opportunities' (Turbin et al., 2014: 171). Turbin and colleagues use of the word 'almost' is probably right, however even if there is 'almost' a secondary labour market in the NHS based on the socio-economic background of the support workforce, this does go some way to explain their treatment compared to registered staff located in the primary labour market.

Are support staff accepted by the NHS – institutional approaches to workforce development

In 2017 Kessler and colleagues published an article in the *Human Resource Management Journal* setting out three stage model associated with the development of new roles in the NHS. In the first stage, which they called 'Emergence', old ways of working dominate, but the initial need for the new role is established. Next comes a 'Legitimacy' stage when the new role begins to be fitted into established structures, processes and systems but only with isolated examples of new ways of working. The old ways still dominate. Finally comes 'Acceptance' when the role is 'taken for granted' and routinely used, (although the authors make the point that roles can stall at the first two stages and not progress to this stage).

Earlier Griffin and colleagues (2010) developed a model to describe the evolution of MSW roles in maternity services. This comprised four-stages:

1. An Initial stage: social, policy, workforce and service pressures result in innovation and pathfinders. The role emerges.
2. A Development stage: initial research on the role is undertaken which results in the identification, and discussion of issues ('making the case').
3. A Consolidation stage: 'hearts and minds' are won; the role is accepted but some issues remain.
4. An Established stage: the role is coherent and consistently defined, career pathways are established, and the role is routinely included in workforce planning. Dedicated training programmes exist.

Whilst these models were developed to explain the incorporation of individual roles within individual employers rather than for the NHS as a whole, they are useful frameworks to consider, more widely, the development of support roles in healthcare. Taking Kessler and colleagues (2017) model and considering the long history of support workers we have charted in this chapter and the last, it could be argued that the period up to the turn of the last century represented an Emergence stage. The roles existed but were frequently contained; suggestions to expand their scope (which challenged the old ways of working which dominated) such as the introduction of the HCA or Assistant Practitioner were contested. It could be argued that following Cavendish (2013), *Talent for Care* (HEE, 2014) and Willis (2015) the support workforce is now entering the Legitimacy stage, with a series of significant developments in the last decade: probably more significant that all the developments of the previous century, with examples of good practice, but also plenty of examples of the old ways of working continuing, including the contesting of support roles as some of the debate about Nursing Associates demonstrated. Discussing the development of support workers in their AHP service a participant in HASKE's (2020) study commented on 'a significant cultural shift' that 'had occurred...whereby an initial resistance...was replaced by acceptance and recognition ... all the staff have been very pleased with what we've done because they could see the potential in these staff' (p. 56). This captures the notion of roles developing in stages. It remains to be seen whether the NHS moves to a full Acceptance stage as far as support workers are concerned.

The Institutional models can be used by individual services to assess to extent to which support workers are fully accepted – or not.

Expansive and restrictive learning cultures

There is evidence that the extent organisation's explicitly or implicitly encourage their staff's development through supportive organisational cultures improves outcomes (see Kyndt et al., 2009 and Gubbins et al., 2012, for example). Learning, though, does not only occur when an employee attends a course or studies for a formal qualification. Learning is embedded (or situated) in an employee's everyday experience of work (Lave and Wenger, 1991). Building on this insight and based on their field work, Fuller and Unwin (2004) considered the barriers and uneven opportunities some employees faced accessing learning at work. In explaining this they identified the importance of how jobs are organised, along with other work processes but also the need to understand the different ways that people learn so as not to 'underplay the role of an individual's background, prior attainments, attitudes, wider experiences and agency' (2004: 138). It is interesting to consider the extent to which this is considered when interventions are introduced for support staff.

One way of explaining this is to draw on Lave and Wenger's (1991) idea of a 'Community of Practice' within workplaces where employees move, when newly employed, from the periphery to a 'fully participating' and 'legitimate' members of the community. Note that these communities do not need to be formally constituted (although the term is used to describe organised learning networks), they could refer to teams or departments or informal groups and relationships at work. An apprentice or student nurse will be seen as peripheral whilst they train to fully acquire the knowledge, skills and behaviours needed for their role. Even after qualifying, they may still be seen as peripheral as they gain experience and orientate to their new workplace and profession. (This touches on the importance of getting on-boarding right, the subject of Chapter 4.)

Given the evidence we have from support workers that they do not always feel valued or feel that they have a voice or are involved in decision making (for example Health Foundation, 2021), it may be the case that they support workers are never perceived as full members of Communities of Practice by their registered colleagues. Support staff may also feel that they do not have agency or high levels of self-efficacy (a malleable concept that refers to the belief that one is able to master or perform a task or overcome a challenge). This compounds the issue of legitimacy as support staff are then denied access to the informal learning that communities provide. Much informal learning is proximal. Lack of access to occupationally relevant qualifications do not help either. This sense of being on the periphery was captured by a radiography Assistant Practitioner – 'The role of AP is a lonely one. You are neither one thing nor another' (quoted in Snaith et al., 2018).

More specifically, Fuller and Unwin (2011) set out facets that typify an expansive workplace culture (restrictive cultures are the converse of these), including:

- Skills are widely distributed amongst the workforce.
- Staff are given time off for learning.
- Staff have access to qualifications.
- The organisation clearly articulates the value of learning.
- There are communities of learning.
- Learning is shared across teams, departments, and agencies.

An audit of the NHS's approach to learning for its support staff such as we have been rehearsing could lead to the conclusion that it demonstrates the features of a restrictive culture (Kessler et al., 2020), for example the lack of CPD funding for unregistered staff. This again could be seen as characteristic of a segmented labour market. We will return to Fuller and Unwin's model in Chapter 5.

Conclusion

This chapter has covered a lot of ground, including bringing the history of the NHS support workforce up to date, briefly reviewing developments in wider UK skills policy, the implications of recent NHS reforms for workforce planning, safe staffing tools and debates as well as insights from a number of academic disciplines that might help explain why support workers have faced long-lasting barriers to their development and why they do not always feel valued.

The aim of this chapter and the last has been to set the scene for the remainder of the book. I have argued that the barriers to full deployment of support staff are not wicked problems, however complex and long-standing they may be – and they are both of those things. There are plenty examples of where organisations get things right for their support staff. 'I would say there has been a significant shift from say 20 years ago when [support workers] were a second pair of hands to actually having their own caseloads' (HASKE, 2020: 51). Allowing support workers to become an extra 'pair of eyes' as well as hands was one of Camilla Cavendish's aims when she reviewed the workforce in 2013. In services like the one the employee just quoted works, doing this delivers benefits for other staff, the support workers themselves and most importantly service users.

Support workers though have not been core to the planning and organisation of healthcare services through much of the history of the NHS (and before). I like the Institutional Model as a way of understanding where the workforce is and the concept of a segmented labour market why it is like it is. Hopefully we are moving to an Acceptance stage, using Kessler and colleagues (2016) term. The Nuffield Trust (2021) called their review of the mental health support workforce 'Untapped'. This phase captures well the consequences of where we are perfectly. Representing a large part of the NHS's workforce many support workers are frustrated that they cannot fully realise their potential. The rest of this book will describe, from pre-employment to pre-registration, how that potential of support workers can be realised.

Checklist

The following checklist is aimed mainly at ICSs, NHS trusts and PCNs. It draws on the guidance I wrote for HEE (2021) to support implementation of their AHP support worker strategy (this strategy is an example of an end-to-end approach to developing the support workforce and one that does address Fuller and Unwin's (2003) call to consider the employee):

1. Undertake a review of the current support workforce. This should comprise data gathering, for example, on turnover rates, age, workforce diversity, titles, qualifications, Job Descriptions, access to formal education, as well as the gathering of the views of support staff themselves. Do they feel valued, what issues matter to them? This book sets out the research evidence about the barriers and issues support workers face, ICS and employer reviews can assess the extent that these are prevalent in a workplace or across a network or system. How are support workers treated compared to other members of staff? The NHS Staff Survey and equality data provide valuable information and benchmarks.

2. Consider establishing a group to plan support workforce development. The group, should be linked into other governance structures and groups, for example, ICS Human Resource Directors, and include support staff and their trade union/professional body representatives. It should review the data gathered and devise an appropriate plan to address issues. For example, it may be the case that the support workforce does not reflect its local population and is also ageing, meaning there is a need for a local recruitment campaign and links with the local employment system could be enhanced. Given that there are likely to be a number of issues to be addressed (because support worker develop-ment is a meta-problem) consider using improvement techniques like Discovery Methodology.

3. Develop a support workforce implementation plan that includes:
    • Measures of improvement. What benefits will result for support workers, other staff, services, and service users? This chapter has identified some of the service-related benefits improving support worker capacity and cap-ability can deliver, future chapters will consider other benefits such as reduced recruitment costs or lower turnover.
    • Consider barriers that need to be overcome and enablers that can assist (such as partnership working).
    • Assigns responsibility for delivery.

4. Identify, share, and build on good practice. An advantage of working across an ICS footprint is that practice in neighbouring NHS trusts and PCNs can be shared. Links can also be made to social care employers.

5. Trust, PCN and ICS boards should consider the recruitment and development of support workers as a matter of routine. Support worker workforce needs should be integrated into wider workforce plans, linked to local population needs.

6. Identify engagement with external employment and skills partners such as colleges and Job Centre Plus.

Note

1 It is worth noting that NVQs were withdrawn in 2015 yet are still being listed as an essen-tial qualification, which would act as a barrier to external recruits or existing NHS staff employed after that date.

References

Addicott, R., Maguire, D., Honeyman, M. and Jabbal. J. (2015). *Workforce Planning in the NHS. The Kings Fund.* Available from: www.kingsfund.org.uk/sites/default/files/field/fie ld_publication_file/Workforce-planning-NHS-Kings-Fund-Apr-15.pdf

Ashwood, L., Macrae, A. and Marsden, P. (2018) Recruitment and retention in general practice nursing: What about pay? *Practice Nurse* 29(2), 83–87.

Augar, P. (2019). *Independent Panel Report to the Post-18 Review of Education and Funding.* Department of Education. Available from: https://assets.publishing.service.gov.uk/gov ernment/uploads/system/uploads/attachment_data/file/805127/Review_of_post_18_ education_and_funding.pdf

Ball, J. and Washbrook, M. (2010). Birthrate Plus: using ratios for workforce planning. *British Journal of Midwifery,* 18(11), pp. 724–731.

Bishop, T. (2008). Healthcare Assistants – an undervalued resource. *Journal of Nurses in General Practice* 36(4), 5.

Bosley, S. and Dale, J. (2008). Healthcare assistants in general practice: practical and conceptual issues if skill-mix change. *British Journal of General Practice* 58(547), 118–124. DOI: 10.3399/bjgp08X277032

Bradley, H. (2015) Gender and work. In *The Sage Handbook of Work and* Employment, edited by Edgell, S., Gottfried, H., and Granter, E. (2015) Sage Publications.

Briggs, A. (1972). *Report of the Committee on Nursing,* Cmnd. 5115. London: HMSO.

Bucan, J., Charlesworth, A., Gershlick, B. and Seccombe, I. (2019) *A Critical Moment: NHS Staffing Trends, Retention and Attrition.* Health Foundation. www.health.org.uk/sites/defa ult/files/upload/publications/2019/A%20Critical%20Moment_1.pdf

Busemeyer, M. R. and Trampusch, C. (2011). *The Political Economy of Collective Skill Formation.* Oxford: Oxford University Press.

Camillus, J. C. (2008). Strategy as a wicked problem. *Harvard Business Review,* May 2008. Available from: https://hbr.org/2008/05/strategy-as-a-wicked-problem

Cavendish, C. (2013). Cavendish Review. An Independent Enquiry into Healthcare Assistants and Support Workers in the NHS and Social Care Settings. London: Department of Health. Available from: https://assets.publishing.service.gov.uk/government/uploads/sys tem/uploads/attachment_data/file/236212/Cavendish_Review.pdf

Charlesworth, A. and Lafond, S. (2017). Shifting from undersupply to oversupply: Does NHS workforce planning need a paradigm shift? *Economic Affairs* 37(1), 36–52.

Department of Education (2021). *Skills for Jobs: Lifelong Learning for Opportunity and Growth.* Available from: www.gov.uk/government/publications/skills-for-jobs-lifelong-learning- for-opportunity-and-growth

Dror, Y. (1971). *Design for Policy Sciences.* New York: Elsevier.

Edwards, M. (1997). The nursing aide: past and future necessity. *Journal of Advanced Nursing* 26, 237–245. DOI: 10.1046/j.1365-2648.1997.1997026237.x

Eidlin, B. (2015). Class and work. In *The Sage Handbook of Work and Employment,* edited by Edgell, S. Gottfried, H. and Granter, E. (2015) Sage.

Fryer, R. (2006). *Learning for a Change.* Department of Health.

Fuller, A. and Unwin, L. (2003). Learning as apprentices in the contemporary UK workplace: Creating and managing expansive and restrictive participation, *Journal of Education and Work* 16(4), 407–426. DOI: 10.1080/1363908032000093012

Fuller, A. and Unwin, L. (2011). Workplace learning and the organisation. In Malloch, M., Cairns, L., Evans, K. and O'Connor, B. N. (eds) in *The Sage Handbook of Learning,* London: Sage.

Griffin, R. (2018). *The Deployment, Education and Development of Maternity Support Workers in England. A Scoping Report to Health Education England*. RCM. Available from: www.rcm. org.uk/media/2347/the-deployment-education-and-development-of-maternity-supp ort-workers-in-england.pdf

Griffin, R. (2020). *A Cost-Benefit Analysis of Enhancing Maternity Support Worker Roles through Utilisation of the Apprenticeship Standard to Implement the Health Education England Maternity Support Worker Competency, Education and Career Development Framework*. King's College London. Available from: https://healtheducationengland.sharepo int.com/Comms/Digital/Shared%20Documents/Forms/AllItems.aspx?id=%2FCo mms%2FDigital%2FShared%20Documents%2Fhee%2Enhs%2Euk%20docume nts%2FWebsite%20files%2FMaternity%2FMSW%20%2D%20Funding%2F04%2E%20 MSW%20Evaluation%2Epdf&parent=%2FComms%2FDigital%2FShared%20Do cuments%2Fhee%2Enhs%2Euk%20documents%2FWebsite%20files%2FMatern ity%2FMSW%20%2D%20Funding

Griffin, R. (2021). *A Rewarding Job, but Frustrating Career. The Education, Development, and Deployment of Clinical Support Workers Employed in NHS Mental Health Services*. London: King's College London.

Griffin, R., Dunkley-Bent, J., Skewes, J. and Linay, D. (2010). Development of maternity support workers in the UK, *British Journal of Midwifery* 18(4), 243–246.

Griffin, R., Blunt, C. and Souster, V. (2013). Building capacity and capability in primary care: A nurse development programme, *Primary Health Care* 21(3), 25–29.

Griffin, R. and Sines, D. (2012). Clinical nursing support workers: Issues and impact, *Nursing Times*, 13 March 2012, 18–19.

Griffiths, P., Nall, J., Drennan, J., Jones, J., Recio-Saucedo, A. and Simon, M., (2014). *The Association between Patient Safety Outcomes and Nurse / Healthcare Assistant Skill Mix and Staffing Levels & Factors that May Influence Staffing Requirements*. University of Southampton. Available from: www.nice.org.uk/guidance/sg1/documents/safe-staffing-for-nursing-in-adult-inpatient-wards-in-acute-hospitals-evidence-review-12

Griffiths, P., Murrells, T., Maben, J., Jones, S. and Ashworth, M. (2010). Nurse staffing and quality of care in UK general practice: Cross-sectional study using routinely collected data. *British Journal of General Practice* 60(570), 36–48. DOI:10.3399/bjgp10x482086

Gubbins, C., Corrigan, S., Garaven, T. N., O'Connor, C., Leahy, D., Long, D. and Murphy, E. (2012). Evaluating a tacit knowledge sharing initiative: A case study, *European Journal of Training and Development* 36(8), 827–847.

Halliday, K., Maskell, G., Beeley, L. and Quick, E. (2020). *Radiology. GIRFT Programme National Speciality Report*. Available from: www.gettingitrightfirsttime.co.uk/wp-cont ent/uploads/2020/11/GIRFT-radiology-report.pdf

HASKE (2020). *The Development of the Allied Health Workforce – An Evaluation for Health Education England*. University of Cumbria.

Health Foundation (2021). Five things we learnt from our work on the health and wellbeing of lower paid NHS staff. (Website) Available from: www.health.org.uk/news-and-comm ent/newsletter-features/five-things-we-learnt-from-our-work-on-the-health-and-wellbe

HEE (2014). *Talent for Care. A National Strategic Framework to Develop the Healthcare Support Workforce*. Available from: www.hee.nhs.uk/sites/default/files/documents/TfC%20Natio nal%20Strategic%20Framework_0.pdf

HEE (2021) *AHP Support Workforce – Grow Your Own Workforce Strategies*. Available from: www. hee.nhs.uk/sites/default/files/documents/AHP_Guide_GYO_Acc.pdf

Hubble, S., Bolton, P. and Lewis, J. (2021). *Further Education Funding in England*. House of Commons Library. Available from: https://researchbriefings.files.parliament.uk/docume nts/CBP-9194/CBP-9194.pdf

Institute of Fiscal Studies (2021). *Education Spending – Further Education and Sixth Forms*. Available from: https://ifs.org.uk/education-spending/Further-Education-and-Sixth-Forms

Jacobs, J. J. (1999). The sex segregation of occupations. In *Handbook of Gender and Work*, edited by Powell, G. N. London: Sage.

Johnson, K. and Moulton, C. (2015) Baseline review: The role of HCAs in general practice. *Practice Nursing* 26(6), 302–305.

Kantaris, X., Radcliffe, M., Acott, K., Hughes, P. and Chambers, M. (2020). Training healthcare assistants working in adult acute inpatient wards in Psychological First Aid: An implementation and evaluation study. *Journal of Psychiatric Mental Health Nursing* 27, 742–751.

Kelley, T. and Kelley, D. (2013). *Creative Confidence. Unleashing the Creative Potential in Us All*. London: William Collins.

Kessler, I., Bach, S., Griffin, R. and Grimshaw, D. (2020). *Fair Care Work. A Post Covid-19 Agenda for Integrated Employment Relations in Health and Social Care*. London: King's College London. Available from www.kcl.ac.uk/business/assets/pdf/fair-care-work.pdf

Kessler, I., Nath, V. and Bach, S. (2016). *The Imagined Futures of Healthcare Support Workers: The Limits of Cultural Influence?* King's College London Paper for the Work, Employment and Society Conference, 6–8 September 2016, Leeds.

Kessler, I., Heron, P. and Spilsbury, K. (2017). Human resource management innovation in health care: The institutionalisation of new support roles. *Human Resource Management Survey* 27(2), 228–245.

Kessler, I. and Heron, P. (2007). NHS modernisation and the role of HCAs. *British Journal of Healthcare Assistants* 4(7), 318–320. https://doi.org/10.12968/bjha.2010.4.7.48906

Kessler, I., Steils, N., Harris, J., Manthorpe, J. and Moriarty, J. (2021). *The Development of the Nursing Associate Role: The Postholder Perspective*. NIHR Policy Research Unit in Health and Social Care Workforce The Policy Institute, King's College London.

Kyndt, E., Dochy, F. and Nijis, H. (2009). Learning conditions for non-formal and informal workplace learning, *Journal of Workplace Learning* 21(5), 369–383.

Lave, J. and Wenger, E. (1991). *Situated Learning. Legitimate Peripheral Participation*. Cambridge University Press.

London South Bank University (2010) *The Impact of Maternity Care Support Workers in NHS Scotland*. *NHS Education for Scotland*. London South Bank University.

Lopes, M. A., Almeida, A. S. and Almada-Lobo, B. (2015). Handling healthcare workforce planning with care: Where do we stand? *Human Resources for Health* 13(1), 38–58.

Neville, S. (2021). NHS England shake-up brings training and technology into health service. *The Financial Times*, 22 November 2021. Available from: www.ft.com/content/5ff19070-a35c-4969-9dc3-c006bef553d2

NHS Confederation (2011). *The Support Workforce in the NHS*. SDO Network Research Digest; 1. NHS Confederation.

NHS Digital (2021). General Practice Workforce, 30 September 2021 – Provisional. Available from: https://digital.nhs.uk/data-and-information/publications/statistical/general-and-personal-medical-services/30-september-2021#

NHS England (2019a). *The NHS Long Term Plan*. Available from: www.longtermplan.nhs.uk

NHS England (2019b). *Interim People Plan*. Available from: www.longtermplan.nhs.uk/wp-content/uploads/2019/05/Interim-NHS-People-Plan_June2019.pdf

NHS England (2021). *2021/22 Priorities and Operational Planning Guidance*. Available from: www.england.nhs.uk/wp-content/uploads/2021/03/B0468-nhs-operational-planning-and-contracting-guidance.pdf

NICE (2022). Safe midwifery staffing for maternity settings. Glossary. Available online at: www.nice.org.uk/guidance/ng4/chapter/5-glossary#acuity

Norris, E. and Adam, R. (2017). *All Change. Why Britain Is So Prone to Policy Reinvention and What Can Be Done About It*. Institute for Government. Available from: www.institutefo rgovernment.org.uk/publications/all-change

Nuffield Trust (2021). *Untapped? Understanding the Mental Health Clinical Support Workforce*. Nuffield Trust. Available from: www.nuffieldtrust.org.uk/research/untapped-understand ing-the-mental-health-clinical-support

O'Dowd, A. (2021). NHS and social care workforce planning is a 'joke' says former health secretary, 25 February 2021, *BMJ* 2021; 372n564.

Palmer, D., Smith, B. and Harris, M. A. (2018). Assistant radiographer practitioners: Creating capacity or challenging professional boundaries? *Radiography* 24(3), 247–251.

Price, R., Miller, L., Hicks, B. and Higgs, A. (2015). The introduction, deployment and impact of assistant practitioners in diagnostic radiography in Scotland, *Radiography* 21, 141–145.

Prime Minister's Office and Department of Health and Social Care (2022). *Build Back Better: Our Plan for Health and Social Care*. Available from: www.gov.uk/government/ publications/build-back-better-our-plan-for-health-and-social-care

RCN (2010). *Assistant Practitioner Scoping Project*. London: RCN Available from: tinyurl. com/RCN-AP-scoping

Richards, M. (2020). *Diagnostics: Recovery and Renewal*. Available from: www.england.nhs. uk/wp-content/uploads/2020/10/BM2025Pu-item-5-diagnostics-recovery-and-rene wal.pdf

Robb, E., Maxwell, E. and Elcock, K. S. (2011). How skill mix affects the quality of care. *Nursing Times* 107(47), 12–13.

Rolewicz, L. and Palmer, B. (2021). The NHS Workforce in Numbers. Facts on staffing and staffing shortages in England. The Nuffield Trust. Available from: www.nuffieldtrust.org. uk/public/resource/the-nhs-workforce-in-numbers

The Shelford Group (n.d.). *Safer Nursing Care Tool Implementation Resource Pack*. Available from: https://dsr.dk/sites/default/files/187/130719_shelford_safer_nursing_final.pdf

Snaith, B., Harris, M.A. and Palmer, D., (2018) A UK Survey exploring the assistant prac- titioner role across diagnostic imaging: current practice, relationships and challenges to progression'. *British Journal of Radiology*, 91 (1091). Available from: www.ncbi.nlm.nih. gov/pmc/articles/PMC6475955/

Spilsbury, K., Adamson, J. Atkin, K., Bloor, K., Carr-Hill, R., McCaughan, D., McKenna, H. and Wakefield, A. (2011). *Evaluation of the Development and Impact of Assistant Practitioners Supporting the Work of Ward-Based Registered Nurses in Acute* NHS (Hospital) Trusts in England. Southampton: National Institute for Health Research. Available from: tinyurl. com/NIHR-Support

Staton, B., Cook, C. and Foster, P. (2021). Does Boris Johnson have the right plan to 'skill up' the UK workforce. *The Financial Times,* 29 September 2021. Available from: www.ft.com/ content/4954c5e0-4592-4dd5-85d3-207657a76afe

Stewart-Lord, A., McLaren, S. M. and Ballinger, S. (2011). Assistant Practitioners' perceptions of the developing role and practice in radiography: Results from a national survey. *Radiography* 17, 193–200.

Teles, S. M. (2013). Kludgeocracy in America. *National Affairs* 17. Available from: www.nati onalaffairs.com/publications/detail/kludgeocracy-in-america

Thornley, C. (2007). Efficiency and equity considerations in the employment of Healthcare Assistants and Support Workers. *Social Policy and Society* 7(2), 147–158.

Turbin, J., Fuller, A. and Wintrup, J. (2014) Apprenticeship and progression in the healthcare sector: Can labour market theory illuminate barriers and opportunities in contrasting occupations? *Journal of Vocational Education & Training* 66(2), 156–174.

United Kingdom Central Council for Nursing Midwifery and Health Visiting (1986). *Project 2000; A New Preparation for Practice.* London: Central Council for Nursing Midwifery and Health Visiting.

Vail, L., Bosley, S., Petrorna, M. and Dale, J. (2011) Healthcare assistants in general practice: a qualitative study of their experiences. *Primary Health Care Research and Development* 12(1), 29–41. DOI: https://doi.org/10.1017/S1463423610000204

Willis, G., Cave, S. and Kunc, M. (2018). Strategic workforce planning in healthcare: A multimethodological approach. *European Journal of Operational Research* 267(1), 250–263.

Willis, P. (2015). Raising the bar: Shape of caring, a review of the future education and training of registered nurses and care assistants. Available from: www.hee.nhs.uk/sites/default/files/documents/2348-Shape-of-caring-review-FINAL.pdf

WRES (2020) Workforce Race Equality Standard. Available from: www.england.nhs.uk/about/equality/equality-hub/equality-standard/

Yao, I., Zhu, X. and Hong, L. (2016). Assessing the midwifery workforce demand: Utilising Birthrate Plus in China. *Midwifery* 42, 61–66.

GROW YOUR OWN APPROACHES TO WORKFORCE DEVELOPMENT

Introduction

Using the *Talent for Care* (HEE, 2014) schema, the remainder of this book's contents are organised around a career cycle that starts with pre-employment, which is described as 'Get Ready', moves to recruitment and initial employment ('Get In'), and then in-work development ('Get On') and ends, for support workers, with access to pre-registration degrees ('Go Further'). From an employer's point of view this approach can be described as a 'Grow Your Own' (GYO) workforce strategy. GYO approaches look to local labour markets, including less traditional labour supply routes to recruit staff, as well as an employer's existing workforce as the key sources for building workforce capacity, capability, and diversity. Recent years have seen a general increase in interest in GYO by employers (Staton, 2022).

A GYO workforce strategy can be further conceptualised as having three distinct but closely linked elements:

- An 'Outside/In' element which seeks to attract and recruit local people from **outside** an organisation **into** NHS it, including from local schools and colleges and residents who may be most distant from the labour market, such as people with disabilities or ex-offenders or the long term unemployed. The role of the NHS as an 'anchor institution', which is discussed in the next chapter, is part of this element (NHS England, 2019).
- An 'In-work development' element that seeks to ensure existing employees have the right knowledge, skills, and behaviours to undertake their roles proficiently working at the top of their scope of practice. This element is also about allowing people develop their careers **within** a role or between roles at the same level, something that can often be neglected as far as NHS support

DOI: 10.4324/9781003251620-5

workers are concerned. Apprenticeships, delegation and appraisals are examples of In-work development GYO interventions. Closely linked to this is ensuring that the factors are in place that constitute good work for example a supportive management culture.

- An 'Inside/Up' element which focuses on creating possibilities for employees already working **inside** an organisation to progress their careers **upwards**. For NHS support workers this could be within different support worker occupations, to a higher support worker grade or into Higher Education. NHS support staff are aspirant, they want to develop their careers and perform their jobs to their best of their ability but too often are unclear of the development opportunities available to them, something that is likely to be true of their managers too (see Griffin, 2021 for example).

GYO is not a new concept as far as the NHS is concerned. In a review, for the Kings Fund, of established GYO interventions adopted by NHS trusts in London in the noughties, Malhotra (2006) concluded that, an 'important factor determining the success of grow-your-own strategies was the degree to which they had become part of mainstream workforce activity: thriving schemes tended to better integrated; less successful ones to be operating in isolation' (p. 22). Malhotra (ibid.) identified four other conditions for success:

1. Organisations explicitly recognised their role in local communities, for example they were actively concerned that their workforce reflected the diversity of those communities *at all levels*. Malhotra described this as 'focused organisational motivation' (ibid., 11).
2. Within organisations there was clear understanding, ownership, and accountability for GYO approaches, so, for example, they engaged not just to key workforce stakeholders but also that they reflected service needs.
3. Strong leadership (including at board level), champions and collaboration were a feature of successful GYO.
4. Effective GYO approaches were measured and evaluated.

Since Malhotra undertook her review, GYO's profile as a specific workforce strategy diminished in the NHS, (although it is a constituent part of other country's healthcare workforce strategies, particularly in Australia). Recent NHS policy documents, such as *The NHS Long Term Plan* (NHS England, 2019) and *Interim People Plan* (NHS England, 2019), made no mention of GYO, for instance. This, though, is changing. It is changing, in part, because of the NHS's growing recognition of its role as an anchor institution (see next chapter) – which was mentioned in *The NHS Long Term Plan* (ibid.), but also because of the NHS's need to address its long-term workforce challenges and ensure employment opportunities are inclusive (Jabbal et al., 2020). In fact, a desire to have a workforce that reflects the communities the NHS serves has, historically, been the main driver for employer's adopting GYO interventions (Malhotra, 2006).

GYO approaches can also help address the workforce shortages amongst registered staff. As we will see in Chapter 7, many support workers would like to progress into registered grades but frequently experience barriers when trying to apply to universities, such as poor access to relevant education and lack of information. Nurses, radiographers, podiatrists, occupational therapists, clinical scientists and midwives drawn from the existing support workforce (via Inside/Up GYO strategies) are more likely to remain working in the NHS trust that they were employed as a support worker in once they graduate (Bateson et al., 2018).

In 2021 the first modern GYO strategy for the NHS was published by HEE, as part of its wider AHP support worker strategy. This document highlighted the ways in which NHS employers could benefit from adopting GYO strategies including by creating a more diverse workforce, but also by reducing staff turnover, creating talent pipelines into the professions, and improving service user satisfaction.

The growing focus on GYO – whether or not interventions are actually described in that way – is also a consequence of the government's wider policy to place greater emphasis on vocational education and training and the NHS's increased engagement with local economic policies.

Whilst each of the GYO elements can be implemented separately, they are best developed as a single workforce strategy, one of Malhotra's (op. cit.) insights ideally at system level. Such an approach creates an *end-to-end* pathway that allows a local resident to join the NHS in an entry-level role and then progress their careers including into pre-registration healthcare degrees.

The following pages describe interventions that can be operationalised by and for support workers at each career stage, starting with 'Get Ready'. Links will be made to the relevant GYO approaches.

References

Bateson, J., Griffin, R., Somerville, M., Hancock, D. and Proctor, S. (2016). *Different People, Different Views, Different Ideas: Widening Participation in Nursing and Radiography Degrees.* Institution of Vocational Learning and Workforce Learning, Bucks New University.

Griffin, R. (2021). *A Rewarding Job, But Frustrating Career. The Education, Development, and Deployment of Clinical Support Workers Employed in NHS Mental Health Services.* King's College London.

HEE (2014) *Talent for Care. A National Strategic Framework to Develop the Healthcare Support Workforce.* Available from: www.hee.nhs.uk/sites/default/files/documents/TfC%20Natio nal%20Strategic%20Framework_0.pdf

HEE (2021) *AHP Support Workforce – Grow Your Own Workforce Strategies.* www.hee.nhs.uk/ sites/default/files/documents/AHP_Guide_GYO_Acc.pdf

Jabbal, J., Chauhan, K., Maguire, D., Randhawa, M. and Dahir, S. (2020). *Workforce Race Inequalities and Inclusions in NHS Providers.* Kings Fund. www.kingsfund.org.uk/sites/defa ult/files/2020-07/workforce-race-inequalities-inclusion-nhs-providers-july2020.pdf

Malhotra, G. (2006). *Grow Your Own. Creating the Conditions for Sustainable Workforce Development*. The Kings Fund. Available from: www.kingsfund.org.uk/sites/default/files/field/field_publication_file/grow-your-own-creating-conditions-sustainable-workforce-development-gita-malhotra-kings-fund-3-august-2006.pdf

NHS England (2019). *The NHS Long Term Plan*. Available from: www.longtermplan.nhs.uk

Staton, B. (2022). UK employers look to hire school leavers as skill shortages bite. *The Financial Times*, 9 January 2022, Available from: www.ft.com/content/5def6c76-4669-4e7c-8a07-b4bd5f153914

PART I
Get ready

3

ENGAGING WITH LOCAL EMPLOYMENT AND SKILLS SYSTEMS

Introduction

For several years I was a member of the West London Alliance (WLA) of local authorities' Employment and Skills Board. I sat alongside representatives from other big West London employers such as Heathrow, HS2 and Transport for London. None though were as big as health and social care in terms of jobs, numbers of buildings, land or procurement. I was struck by how normal it was for these employers to engage with their colleges or schools or specialist employment agencies, in order to encourage local people to work for them. At the time (2016–2019) the West London economy was booming and there was a shortage of labour. The NHS in West London was competing with employers, like Heathrow, for staff yet had very minimal engagement with the area's employment system and was not actively seeking to recruit local people. This changed (largely in response to the wider economic impact of Covid-19, as discussed below). As an aside, I was also struck by the clarity by which the other employers were able to articulate their skills needs, something the NHS seemed to struggle to do.

The subject of this chapter is labour supply – how and where the future NHS support workforce will be recruited from. The focus is on the role of an underutilised, (by the NHS), supply route – local labour markets. Put simply, labour markets are where people find jobs and where employees recruit employees. *Local* labour markets comprise jobs available in a locality (for example in an area covered by an ICS), and employers based in that area (like a hospital or general practice surgery or care home). This is the demand side of a local labour market. Potential recruits, who represent the supply-side of the market, live in that area. They may be studying in a local school or college, be working for another employer (based in the area or outside) or be unemployed or economically inactive. A large number of

DOI: 10.4324/9781003251620-7

organisations in addition to employers participate in local labour markets including, in particular, colleges and local authorities.

In GYO terms this chapter is concerned with Outside/In GYO approaches – interventions aimed at bringing people from outside the NHS into employment. The first step in this approach is raising awareness of the massive number of jobs available in the NHS. This is no mean feat. 'The issue, especially for the NHS is not just increasing the numbers [of young people wishing to enter heath careers] but also to widen the view of the jobs available in the healthcare sector' (Employers and Education, 2018a: 17). Interventions such as Ambassadors, job shadowing and work experience, alongside working with partners such as colleges will raise awareness of NHS job opportunities including those available in support roles. What is needed, but has historically been lacking, is a deliberate decision to promote support worker roles as a career. This could also help address shortages of registered staff if comprehensive GYO approaches are followed. Someone recruited as a Footcare Assistant could, for example, be supported to progress into a podiatry degree to become a podiatrist for example. The fact that they were recruited from a local labour market means that are more likely to remain working in the area, even when they become a registered professional.

The benefits of Outside/In GYO approaches go beyond capacity building.

> The NHS provides better care when the people employed in its services reflect the diversity of the communities it serves. A more diverse workforce brings a broader range of experience to services and demonstrates to members of individual communities that they are valued and respected. Moreover, research tells us that good employment itself improves people's health outcomes and the NHS has an important role as an anchor institution within communities to promote and expand the diversity of employment.
>
> *Learning Disability Employment Programme, 2022*

Ensuring the NHS workforce better reflects the communities it serves adds social value and community wealth (The Centre for Local Economic Strategies, 2016). Moreover, employment is also a key social determinant of health and well-being (Health Foundation, 2018), so an Outside/In GYO approach further helps address health inequalities, particularly when those who are furthest from the labour market are supported into work.

The NHS is an institution whose activities touch on many parts of local economies, but perhaps in respect of employment, education and training more than any other area. 'As a major employer the NHS has a role to play in being more influential and proactive' locally (NHS Confederation and The Future College Commission, 2020: 28). A way for the NHS to achieve this is through engagement with local economic strategies, which are led by local authorities. Local economic strategies seek to bring together private and public sector partners to support local development and growth, including for those citizens, communities, and groups who are most distant from the labour market. The latest iteration of local economic strategies, in respect of skills, is the creation of *Local Skills Improvement Boards* and *Plans*.

Those employers I sat alongside on the West London Employment and Skills Board understood the importance of recruiting local people into their organisations, as well as the wider benefits that accrued from collaborating with employment (and skills) partners, such as colleges, Job Centre Plus and local authorities. My reflection was that too often the NHS looks inwards rather than outwards. This is changing. The enhanced role of ICS in workforce planning is a critical development in helping the NHS look outwards to engage with local labour markets. Outside/In GYO could become a key strategy for recruiting support staff. We will start by thinking about who individual NHS employers and ICSs should be working with.

Local labour market organisations and how to find them

Interventions associated with Outside/In GYO approaches require working in collaboration with a potentially large number of agencies and institutions (Health Foundation, 2018). Supporting young people with disabilities into NHS employment, to take one Outside/In GYO intervention as an example requires working with the following organisations: education settings (schools and colleges), national employment agencies like DFN Project Search, local authority Special Education, Education and economic teams, specialist employment agencies, voluntary organisations, and coaches, as well as the young people themselves.

HEE (2021) listed the potential local labour market partners:

- Schools.
- Colleges.
- Universities.
- Independent Training Providers.
- Local authorities.
- Job Centre Plus.
- Employment Support agencies.
- Faith organisations.
- The voluntary sector.
- Charitable organisations.
- Community groups.
- Prisoner and offender centres.
- Veteran organisations.
- Immigration and detention centres.
- Probation services.

Working with many of these agencies will not only help secure future labour supply, deliver efficiencies and savings on recruitment costs, but also create partnerships that can help deliver other aspects of support worker – and indeed other staff's – employment and development, such as apprenticeships and progression into pre-registration degrees.

There are, though, a lot of potential partners and some compete with each other. A significant challenge for labour market organisations on both the supply and demand sides is dealing with this complexity and fragmentation (The Centre for Local Economic Strategies, 2016). There is an additional and related problem for labour market organisations, like colleges, who want to work with the NHS – who do you speak too? Assessing why the NHS and colleges have not worked more closely together the NHS Confederation and The Future College Commission (2020) noted that, from a college's point of view, (and no doubt other organisations too), 'the scale of the NHS can be daunting' (p. 12). Their solution was to create 'navigator' roles. Such roles can also be described as 'system integrators'. The role's purpose is to engage and connect partners, acting as a contact point so there is 'one front door' into sectors (NHS Confederation and The Future College Commission, 2020). A 'navigator' role could be employed at a systems level. That is essentially what I was doing in West London and why I sat on the WLA's Employment and Skills Board. It is all about joining the dots up. *Local Skills Improvement Plans* also provide the opportunity for the NHS to engage with local labour markets. Local authority economic teams are most likely to have contacts with all the key partners in the local employment and skills system. Doing so will assist the NHS to play a more active role as an 'anchor institute' in its local communities.

The NHS's role as an anchor institution and its contribution to community wealth

Tucked away at the very end of *The NHS Long Term Plan* (NHS England, 2019), in its last paragraph in fact, is an important statement. The *Plan* says that the NHS, acting as an anchor institution, 'creates social value in local communities' (p. 120). Social value refers to the difference that an organisation (or activity) can make to the community it is located in, but what are anchor institutions?

The Centre for Local Economic Strategies (2021) defines anchor institutions as organisations that have

> an important presence in a place, usually through a combination of being large scale employers, and/or as the largest purchasers of goods and services in a locality, or through controlling large areas of land [and/or] having relatively fixed assets. [Such] organisations are tied to a particular place by their mission, histories, physical assets and local relationships.

Examples of anchor institutions include local authorities, universities, trade unions, football and rugby league clubs[1] and large local businesses.

Applying the Centre for Local Economic Studies' definition to the NHS it is clear why it is a significant anchor institution with a major role to play in its communities beyond providing healthcare services, even if that role has not been well understood or developed in the past (Health Foundation, 2018; Edwards, n.d. and Institute of Government, 2020):

- In many localities the NHS will be the largest single employer.
- Nationally the NHS owns 6.9 million hectares of land.
- The NHS procures £70 billion worth of goods and services a year including the commissioning of education, not least the £200 million a year NHS apprenticeship levy in 2021.
- NHS staff and service users are major users of local services including transport.

Michael Wood is in the NHS Confederation's Head of Health Economic Partnerships and has long promoted the role that healthcare organisations can play in their local communities. 'Often', he told me,

> the NHS doesn't realise just how much it matters to local communities, both economically and socially. This is particularly the case in terms of employment and skills where we will be the largest employer in every locality. Realising the potential of an 'anchor' means reflecting on how, where, and why we recruit. Are we inspiring people, raising ambition and supporting social mobility? Are we trying to improve the health of the population or simply fill vacancies? These are the questions that more and more NHS Trusts are rightly asking themselves.

Focusing on the impact that acting as an anchor institution can have in respect of employment – the subject of this chapter – it is clear why *The NHS Long Term Plan* (NHS England, 2019) signalled the importance of this role. This is a 'win–win'. The NHS needs to recruit staff, with many of its vacancies in entry-level jobs such as clinical support worker roles. In West London, the NHS with social care employers together had 12,000 entry-level vacancies – each year.

Employment is a key factor influencing individual health and well-being (Goodman, 2016; Health Foundation, 2018). Economic factors, such as in-work poverty and unemployment are significant social determinants of health (Health Foundation, 2021a). It is estimated that only 20–30% of health is derived from the formal provision of care, with the majority being determined by wider social factors such as employment, pollution and housing (NHS Confederation and The Future College Commission, 2019). Prior to the Covid-19 pandemic, health inequalities were estimated to cost NHS hospitals £4.8 billion each year (Asari et al., 2016). By actively and deliberately seeking to recruit local people into work the NHS can not only address staff shortages but also contribute to reducing health inequalities, particularly when strategies support those who face barriers to employment, such as people with disabilities.

It should also be noted here that in addition to its role as an employer, the NHS can also make a significant contribution to population health as a commissioner of education and training. Access to education also matters to individual health, because learning 'provides the skills, attributes, and specialist knowledge needed to secure good jobs and participate in society – building blocks of a healthy life' (Health Foundation, 2021b: 4). By the time a person is 30 years of age if they have only acquired the lowest level of educational attainment, they will have a life expectancy that is four years lower than someone who has attained the highest level. Education boosts employment and earnings – throughout an individual's lifetime and this in turn 'has the potential to improve health and reduce health inequalities within the population' (ibid., 9).

So far we have considered who the NHS needs to work with locally to help deliver GYO Outside/In workforce shortages and the benefits of doing so. The rest of this chapter will set out the practical interventions that can be utilised to attract local people into support worker employment. A key step in this approach is ensuring that people – young people studying at school or college, people who may be unemployed or economically inactive or adults considering a career change – are aware of the opportunities that the NHS has, so that they can judge whether working as a healthcare assistant is right for them and if it is how to they can access NHS jobs (which is not always straightforward).

How to raise awareness of NHS careers

Young people studying at school or college are a key source of future labour supply for the NHS – either as graduates or as direct-entry employees; this is why engagement with education settings to provide careers information and advice is so important. A survey by CBI/Pearson's in 2019 found that 95% of employers had links with secondary schools and 91% with colleges. These links had been made, firstly, to aid recruitment through the provision of careers information, advice and guidance (82%), but also to support apprenticeship delivery (73%) or to offer work experience (69%). A survey in 2022 by the Institute of Student Employers, found that nearly a quarter (23%) of companies planned to 'rebalance' the proportion of young people they recruited, towards college and school leavers. This was partly driven by the apprenticeship levy and a desire to recruit into apprenticeships to utilise the fund, but also by a desire to recruit young people with specific vocational training.

Statistics for the extent of the NHS's engagement with schools and colleges is not available; however, it is probable that it is less extensive than CBI/Pearsons' (op. cit.) recorded for employers generally. Evidence for this is the relatively low number of Ambassadors (discussed below) in the NHS and the degree of awareness of NHS careers amongst young people. When asked what careers were available in the NHS, young people named just five occupations – out of the 350 available. These were – nursing, midwifery, medical, dental and physiotherapy (Education and Employment, 2018b). Many NHS occupations it would appear are invisible to school and college students. In a 2019 editorial for the *Radiography* journal, which discussed the shortage of therapeutic radiographers, the editor lamented the lack of awareness about the profession amongst the general public and wrote that getting 'the message out … about our role is vitally important to ensure the future of thera-peutic radiographers' (p. 1).

'Getting the message out' is a key challenge for the NHS nationally and locally. How do you make people aware of the multitude of occupations the NHS has to offer? It is hard to think of a role that cannot be undertaken somewhere in the health service. Pilot? Yes – air ambulance. Chef? Yes – catering roles. Computing? Yes – the NHS is one of the largest employers of IT skills in the UK. Gardeners, artists, musicians (art and music therapy), actors (dramatherapy), finance, administration, and so on and so on. When giving career talks, I used to ask the audience to try to think of a job that you could not undertake in the NHS. Outside astronaut, train driver and lifeguard (I decided hydrotherapy did not count), they and I were hard pressed to come up with one.

It is also unlikely that many people, prior to joining healthcare employment, are aware of the difference between registered and unregistered roles, and consequently that it is possible to work in a patient-facing role as part of a nursing, midwifery or AHP team, earning reasonable pay, with good terms and conditions, without having to go to university or that there are apprenticeship-based routes into the registered professions that mean people can train to be a nurse or midwife or whatever whilst still earning and being employed as a support worker.

Increasing awareness of possible NHS careers is only part of what is needed, though. Young people and adults alike need to be convinced to work in healthcare. Of those five professions that had a profile amongst young people, only 5% of the young people in the study wanted to become doctors, 2% nurses and 0.5% dentists, midwives, or physiotherapists (Education and Employment, 2018b). What factors might deter people from working in a healthcare role? The process starts young. 'Career aspirations are set early' (Rogers et al., 2020: 8) with family members playing a prominent role. Nearly three-quarter (59%) of 7–11-year-olds, who have made a preferred career choice had that choice shaped by their parents, guardians or other family member. Less than 1% had heard directly about the career they were interested in from someone working in that role or from that industry (Education and Employers, 2018b).

BOX 3.1 RAISING AWARENESS OF NHS CAREERS AMONGST YOUNG PEOPLE – *STEP INTO THE NHS*

Step into the NHS is a web-based careers resource aimed at primary and secondary schools. It seeks to raise awareness of the breadth of NHS careers through case studies and video stories, as well as providing information on apprenticeships and resources for teachers to use at Key Stage 2, 3 and 4. An annual competition is also run. The site includes a quiz for young people to complete which leads to suggestions about possible career choices in healthcare. (I completed it and the results suggested I think about becoming a psychiatrist, which to be fair, is not an unappealing suggestion.)

Choices made at primary school can be hard to dislodge in later years. By the age of 15 years old, most young people have a set view of what career they would like to pursue – and those they do not want too. It is probable that career interventions, such as career talks, at a later age for school students are not that effective. 'Very few 17- and 18-year olds describe career advisors as an influence on their career choices (10%)' (Rogers et al., 2020: 8). It would also seem though that very few older school children have experienced a talk about possible careers from a visiting speaker, perhaps as few as 11% (ibid.).

Whether to challenge stereotypes, which discourage young people joining certain careers because they do not think they are for them, or to raise awareness about opportunities and prospects in terms of careers information, advice and guidance, it is important for employers to intervene as early as primary school (HEE, 2015). 'Early intervention can be a very effective targeted way of raising children's aspirations and broadening their horizons' (Education and Employers, 2018a: iv).

Rogers and colleagues (2020) point to the importance of children as young as seven years old hearing about potential future jobs from employees and the particular value of employers engaging with the young people's educational activities. Rogers and colleagues report that it is 'important to give employer encounters the best chance of a "lightbulb moment" with young people – this is partly about volume (you don't know what you don't know until you see it) and partly linking encounters explicitly into pathway reflection, iterative research and decision-making. What makes employer engagement special is that it…[focuses] on broadening horizons and raising aspirations, giving children a wide range of experiences of the world including the world of work' (p. 15). The *Step into the NHS* website (see Box 3.1 above) includes resources for teachers, including those in primary school.

One barrier to attracting people into healthcare roles can be stereotypes about those roles. Stereotyping can mean that 'choices are limited by … gender, ethnicity or socio-economic background' (Rogers et al., 2020: 14). This can be a particular challenge in healthcare. 'Children's aspirations appear to be shaped by gender-specific ideas about certain jobs…Conceptions of traditional feminity, specifically around "nurturing" or "caring" roles, may explain the difference between the number of girls wanting to be a teacher or doctor compared to boys' (Employers and Education, 2018b: iv). Again, this starts young. Research shows that 'by the time they start primary school, children are already starting to form taxonomies of adult roles' (Education and Employers and HEE, 2021: 11). The comparatively low incidence of men within the nursing profession, which is an international phenomenon, is a clear example of this (see Kluczynska, 2016 for example).

Misconceptions about health careers can go even beyond this type of stereotyping. A literature review by Glerean and colleagues (2017), investigating young people's attitude towards a career in nursing, found an outdated and negative perception of the profession as one characterised by poor working conditions, shift work and low levels of autonomy. Nursing was also perceived as being inferior to the role of doctors in terms of the care provided to patients. The educational demands required on nursing and potential developmental pathways were poorly understood. These perceptions were again shaped by families, friends and the media.

Turning to the evidence about the factors that *attract* people into healthcare careers, Wu and colleagues (2015) undertook a literature review of international peer reviewed studies that investigated the reasons why degree students had chosen careers in medicine, nursing, pharmacy and dentistry. They found that these decisions were shaped by four drivers:

1. Intrinsic factors such as a desire to help others.
2. Extrinsic factors such as such as financial reward and professional prestige.
3. Socio-economic factors, for example stereotyping (that some professions are female dominated, for example, which deterred men from applying).
4. Interpersonal factors such as the influence of family members.

Based on the evidence, they argued that different attraction factors impact differently in different professions, a point also identified by Sok and colleagues (2017). For example, a *personal* interest in health care was an important reason why people chose a nursing or dental career but was less important for pharmacists. Ten Hoeve and colleagues (2017) also found that the main reasons students had chosen to study to become nurses were (1) the caring aspects of the role, (2) previous experience of healthcare, (3) the impact of role models and (4) the availability of job opportunities.

For radiography, both Vosper and colleagues (2005) and Bamba and colleagues (2013) found the reason people were attracted to the profession was that it provided not only an opportunity to work with, and help, people (as in the cases of nursing and dentistry) but also the opportunity to work with technology. The radiography profession was perceived as 'working in healthcare but not medicine/nursing' (Vosper et al., 2015: 83).

This evidence – which focuses on choices individuals made to join healthcare degrees and subsequently registered roles rather than support worker careers – points to the fact that a 'one-size fits all' approach to careers information may be less effective than targeted approaches based on what is known about attraction factors and also the importance of challenging perceptions about roles. Whilst there are few studies on the reasons why people chose to become support workers, it is reasonable to assume that their motivation is similar to choices made to become a registered professional.

BOX 3.2 WHAT ACTIVITIES ARE SUCCESSFUL IN RAISING AWARENESS OF CAREERS?

While evidence is not extensive on the impact of specific interventions designed to raise awareness about careers and attract young people into them, including healthcare ones, job shadowing, work experience, mentoring and work-related educational activity (like projects) have 'generally positive outcomes' (Education and Employers Research, 2018a: 15). A study of secondary school children by Mann and Dawkins (2014) found over half (58%) thought work experience effective, around 35% competitions, 34% mock interviews, 33% career talks, 32% work visits and 31% mentoring. Whatever approaches are adopted, it is essential employers and education settings work closely together and frequently to raise young people's awareness of careers, their aspirations and providing them with work related knowledge, experience and skills (Education and Employers, 2018b; Rogers et al., 2020).

Whilst we have only been able to touch briefly on the factors that shape people's career choices, the key points are:

(1)   That there is a need to raise awareness of the very broad range of jobs available in the NHS, including support worker ones.
(2)   That there is a need to engage with young people from when they are in primary schools and to do so frequently.
(3)   Stereotypes need to be challenged. The main way that the NHS has sought to engage with education settings is through so-called Ambassadors.

NHS Ambassadors

The *NHS Ambassadors* scheme was formally launched in 2018 (Education and Employers and HEE, 2021), although NHS ambassadors existed prior to that. One of the recommendations of *Talent for Care* (HEE, 2014) was that greater use should be made of ambassadors. Ambassadors are health care workers, including support workers, who talk to children and young people about their jobs and the NHS more widely (HEE, 2015). In a review undertaken in 2021 it was found that 4,511 NHS staff had acted as ambassadors, undertaking a range of activities, including career talks, acting as reading partners, delivering subject specific talks and participating in 'career speed dating' events (ibid.). The later refers to NHS staff from a range of occupations (or with other employers) describing their roles to young people individually or in groups. Young people move from table to table.

BOX 3.3 THE BENEFITS OF NHS AMBASSADORS

A review of the *NHS Ambassador* scheme, and evidence more generally, identified a series of benefits arising from ambassador schemes for employees, employers and education settings alike (Education and Employers and HEE, 2021):

- The learning of a new skill–reported by 81% of NHS Ambassadors.
- Perceptions by staff who volunteered as NHS Ambassadors that they were more productive and efficient at work as a result of the volunteering.
- Young people gained a more informed view of NHS careers. After one event for example, 27% *more* young people felt that being an AHP was a valid career choice, than had done so prior to it.

- Young people learnt about a wider range of NHS roles through interaction with NHS Ambassadors. Amongst primary school children 75% said they had learnt about at least one new role following an interaction with a NHS Ambassador and 86% of secondary school children had.
- Meeting a NHS Ambassador led to 16% of young people to change their minds about their career choices.

As we will see *NHS Ambassadors,* though, are not the only way that the NHS can raise awareness of job opportunities. Other interventions include career events, work experience, mentoring, volunteering and job shadowing. Before these are considered the benefits of the NHS working more closely with colleges, which have been described as 'engines of social mobility and inclusion' (Augar, 2017: 118), will be considered. •

The importance of working with colleges

The Further Education (FE) sector comprises local authorities, colleges, independent training providers (ITPs), charities and employers that deliver state funded education to people aged 16 years old or over (with the exception of universities or schools). This section focuses on colleges, the largest providers of FE. The reason for this is that colleges have an important, but underdeveloped role (particularly compared to universities), to play in securing the future NHS support workforce. Unpublished research conducted in North West London in 2018, found that only a quarter of local college students studying a healthcare vocational qualification entered either health or social care employment.

> In discussions with college leaders, it is often cited that the NHS can be perceived as something of a passive employer, overly reliant on universities and not fully aware of, or prepared to maximise, the opportunities to grow a local workforce through the wider skills system ... colleges are the main link for the NHS to recruit in the communities it serves, opening up opportunity to a much greater and diverse pool of talent and increasing the ability to retain and further develop its workforce.
>
> *NHS Confederation and The Future College Commission, 2019: 13*

There are at least six reasons why the NHS should work more closely with colleges-

1. Colleges teach healthcare vocational qualifications, such as Higher Nationals and Technical Levels, to 350,000 students, 71% of whom are women and who have an average age of 31 years old (NHS Confederation and The Future College Commission, 2019). Some 650,000 college students are also studying a Science, Technology, Engineering, or Mathematics subject (Association

of Colleges, 2020), and will have knowledge relevant to a number of NHS occupations. All these students represent a large pool of potential future NHS support and other staff. Colleges, as a result, should be 'seen more as recruitment partners' than they currently are (NHS Confederation and The Future College Commission, 2019: 14).

2. Colleges teach a large number of social care qualifications and can therefore 'play an important role in supporting the closer integration of health and social care' (NHS Confederation and The Future College Commission, 2019: 10).

3. College students are a source of recruits not only into support worker roles, but also into healthcare degrees including for shortage professions – if they are aware of them.

4. In addition to teaching young people colleges have an important role re-training and re-skilling adults and assisting people distant from the labour market, such as the long term unemployed (Augar, 2017).

5. College students tend to be more representative of local communities, than university graduates are. Widdowson and King (n.d.) point out that colleges are more likely to be embedded in their local communities than universities. This point was echoed by the Augar (2017) review – '[c]olleges are often very long established and deeply embedded in their communities' (p. 118). FE programmes help address economic, social and health inequalities including support for people whose first language may not be English (NHS Confederation and The Future College Commission, 2019).

6. Colleges deliver education programmes from RQF level 1 to foundation degrees and beyond that can benefit *existing* employees, including the provision of apprenticeships and functional skills – which may be free to students and employers.

Despite these benefits, engagement between colleges and the NHS historically has not been well developed. According to The NHS Confederation and The Future College Commission (2019) review, there are a number of reasons for this:

- Lack of clarity about who it is best to engage with in either sector.
- Lack of understanding about each sector.
- A tendency for any engagement that does take place to do so in silos rather than through sustained engagement.
- Regular changes in personnel make building long term relations challenging.
- Higher Education is held in greater esteem by the NHS than FE.
- There is a lack of understanding of the breadth of careers available in the NHS.
- There is no stability in terms of funding.
- Colleges may be in competition with each other as well as with private education providers.

How to address this? The discussion above about anchor institutions pointed to the important role of ICSs in helping to engage with colleges and the FE sector more generally, along with the benefit of creating 'navigator' or 'integrator' roles. In addition, greater collaboration could also be achieved through the following initiatives:

- Colleges could invite ICS/NHS employer leaders to visit them, see their facilities and meet their students.
- College representatives could be included on ICS People Boards (many of which will have university's represented).
- Colleges could be included in individual programmes of work.
- The creation of an ICS-level group that brings the NHS, FE and HE together (see box below).

BOX 3.4 HIGHER EDUCATION AND FURTHER EDUCATION WORKING TOGETHER

In response to the economic impact of Covid-19 on the local economy, local authorities in West London developed an economic recovery plan. In this the NHS was formally recognised as a key partner not only in developing the strategy itself but also as a key growth sector with a significant role to play in supporting the delivery of the strategy. The North West London ICS, in turn, recognised the role local authorities and other partners could play in meeting its need to recruit at pace the workforce required to staff the mass vaccination centres (see next chapter), but also how collaboration could help ensure Covid-19 did not widen existing inequalities.

As part of their recovery strategy, West London local authorities bought the universities and colleges in the area together that had an interest in health and social care in a group, along with representatives of the ICS. The joint group was an opportunity to discuss areas of common concern, access funding (by successfully bidding together for London Mayor Adult Education funds for training and to research why the majority of college students studying healthcare vocational qualifications did not enter healthcare employment) and to agree a progression agreement to allow sufficiently qualified FE students' progress into healthcare degrees.

Vocational qualifications – Technical Levels

FE has a long history of delivering specialist work-related qualifications, including for people interested in a career in healthcare. From 2021, young people in England had two main options for post 16 study – A levels or Technical (T) Levels. T Levels are replacing the vast majority of Business and Technology Education Council (better known as BTEC) qualifications, but like them combine practical learning with theory and subject relevant learning.

T Levels, last for two years and their content comprises 80% classroom teaching and 20% industry placement. In terms of academic rigour, they are equivalent to A levels. The top T Level grades ('Distinction★' and 'Distinction') are equal to A Level – AAA★ and AAA and therefore T Levels should be recognised by universities, indeed a previous Secretary of State for Education said the government's aspiration was for them to become a 'gold standard' qualification (Parker, 2021).

T Levels have three components:

1. A RQF level 3 Technical Qualification.
2. Level 2 functional skills (digital skills are also taught).
3. Industry placements of approximately 45 days spread over two years. Placements can be organised as a series of day releases or blocks of time. They can be shared between employers in a sector, so that, for example, employers, including primary care and social care ones, within an ICS footprint (or beyond) could come together to offer placements, thereby reducing the capacity challenge for individual employers.

There are three T Levels that are relevant for people who might be interested in a healthcare career:

- Health.
- Healthcare Science.
- Science.

BOX 3.5 THE ADULT EDUCATION BUDGET (AEB)

The AEB is a government set budget that funds the education (excluding apprenticeships) and learning support delivered by the FE sector for adults with low skill attainment, who are in receipt of low pay or who are unemployed. Funding includes functional skills training. Depending on eligibility learners on AEB courses either have their full training costs covered or co-fund.

Funding is also available for disadvantaged groups who may require additional support including for their wellbeing. There are rules in respect of who is entitled for full or co-funded learning based on age, employment status and existing qualifications. Around 50% of the national AEB has been devolved to the six Mayoral Combined Authorities including London and Greater Manchester (although traineeships remain a national programme).

The Health T Level comprises a core component that all students study and then five specialist pathway options which students chose one of. Together this provides students with the relevant knowledge and skills to either work in healthcare (in a support role) or to apply for a higher healthcare qualification such as a foundation degree or undergraduate degree.

The shared core component comprised in 2022 the following modules-

1. Working within the health and science sector.
2. The healthcare sector.
3. Health, safety and environmental regulations in the health and science sector.
4. Health and safety regulations applicable in the healthcare sector.
5. Managing information and data within the health and science sector.
6. Managing personal information.
7. Good scientific and clinical practice.
8. Providing person–centred care.
9. Health and wellbeing.
10. Infection prevention and control in health specific settings.
11. Saf5 eguarding.

The five specialist modules were:

1. Adult nursing.
2. Midwifery.
3. Mental health nursing.
4. Care of children and young people.
5. Therapy.

Assessment is through written examinations and an employer-set project.

T Levels create the opportunity for NHS employers to work much more closely with colleges in a number of ways. This can be done through:

- Shared teaching, placements and employer set assignments which are an opportunity to provide potential recruits with experience of roles, including those that they may be less aware of (such as the smaller AHP occupations), as well as a taste of the reality of healthcare work.
- The potential of co-delivery. Outside of the placements there is scope for NHS staff to design and deliver classroom teaching. This is particularly important when colleges do not employ lecturers with specific professional clinical expertise.
- Involvement in the recruitment of T Level students, which is an opportunity to highlight NHS career opportunities. T Levels should be incorporated into any education setting's engagement strategy,

To be effective employers need to work with colleges to ensure T Levels can be implemented successfully.

Other opportunities working with colleges

In addition to training future NHS employees, there are other reasons why healthcare employers should work more closely with colleges:

- Colleges deliver a range of technical, employment and work focused qualifications (Leavey, 2021). These span from RQF level 1 to foundation degrees and beyond. In fact, around 10% of higher education provided in England (to a total of 137,000 people) is delivered in 200 colleges. Colleges also teach apprenticeships.
- Colleges can design and deliver bespoke learning for NHS employers. Working with NHS employers in the North East of England a college developed training to support staff to deal with distressing situations (case study quoted in NHS Confederation and The Future College Commission, 2019).
- Colleges deliver formal functional skills training which is free for adults who do not have GCSE English or Mathematics at grade 9-4 or A-C.
- Working together with universities and employers, colleges can be central to developing progression agreements that aim to widen participation into pre-registration degrees. Progression agreements are formal arrangements between universities and colleges (and ITPs) that allow vocational students, which can include apprentices, to access specific degrees. Normally a college student passing a vocational qualification would be guaranteed an interview for a university course. Progression agreements also allow partners to address any barriers to progression (like student confidence or study skills).

BOX 3.6 THE NHS AND COLLEGES WORKING TOGETHER: SURGE CARE ASSISTANTS

In 2021 in response to the pressures on ward staff caused by the second Covid-19 surge, including the redeployment of staff, Imperial College Healthcare NHS Trust worked with their local colleges (West London College and Harrow and Uxbridge College) to create a new role, called a Surge Care Assistant (SCA). The aim of the SCA role was to carry out routine tasks on the ward, such as changing bed linen, helping patients to eat and drink, assisting patients to sit or stand and supporting personal care. Healthcare BTEC students studying at the colleges in the final year of their course aged 18 years old or over filled the role on a four-week placement. Both colleges cleared the students' study calendar so that they could work full time as SCAs during their placement. The students worked in pairs, one covering an early shift and the other the late shift.

The trust's Head of Learning, Sharon Probets, explained that 'the need for additional staff during the second surge made it possible to train health &

care student from our local college and have them on paid placement for four weeks to support ward teams with basic patient care. The success of those placements means we are now building a Technical Level placement programme for health & care students.'

Adult career changers

Students studying in colleges and schools are one source of the future NHS support and registered workforce. There are though others, which we will consider in this section: adult career changers and people who experience barriers to employment, such as ex-offenders or people with disabilities. These routes have been less frequently used by the NHS but are more common internationally. An international shortage of nurses has resulted in dedicated campaigns and programmes to support adult career changers move into the profession in countries such as the United States.

The NHS has rarely considered the potential of adult career changers, as a source of labour. An exception was the campaign run by HEE in 2021 to encourage career changers to join the AHPs (HEE, 2021). This campaign highlighted the very broad range of jobs some AHPs had prior to joining the NHS, including in publishing, law, music, a tool setter, restaurant management, the civil servants, project management, food technology, the armed forces and computing to name a few, along with the fact the many had transferable skills. There has also for some time been a structured programme to assist Armed Forces personnel who leave the services to join the NHS (see Box 3.7). These, though, are the exception and the NHS has lacked a coherent career changer strategy such as teaching has for example (DfE, 2019).

As a result, there is a paucity of evidence on why people might choose to change careers in order to work for the NHS and what needs to be done to facilitate that change. It is probable that insights drawn from research about people who career change to become teachers hold some insights for the NHS. A decision to switch careers and train to be a teacher 'is closely related to the desire to find more fulfilling and rewarding work' (Williams, 2013: 48). It is likely that the factors attracting career changers to a new career are no different to those that attract people who chose it as their first employment (ibid.). The fact, as we have already discussed, that awareness of the broad range of NHS careers is low and there may be misconceptions about the nature of healthcare work, means that many people who might be interested in working in a healthcare role are simply not aware of the options. The spotlight Covid-19 placed on the NHS and the consequent increase in interest in working for it would seem to endorse this. Career changers represent a potential source of future NHS workers, including support workers. As many as 40% of people in work intend to quit their current role and work elsewhere (De Smet et al., 2021). An advantage of employing career changers as a supply of labour is that they are work-ready with many transferable skills including lived experience of caring, trades, information technology skills and communications.

BOX 3.7 STEP INTO HEALTH

Not to be confused with *Step Into the NHS* (see Box 3.1 above), *Step Into Health* is a programme run by NHS Employers, in partnership with the Armed Forces, that has two aims. Firstly it seeks to raise awareness amongst Forces personnel of NHS careers, and secondly to make NHS organisations aware of the transferable skills that those personnel have (such as leadership, management, team working and communications skills). Links are made into the Forces' transition programme to match potential recruits with vacancies.

Whilst under researched evidence suggests that a significant number of the people who wish to change careers, might like to move into the NHS jobs.[2] The National Careers Service (Box 3.8) in London report that the NHS was the organisation most frequently mentioned by the over 90,000 people they supported during the year, but, tellingly, potential career changers were unsure of the routes into NHS employment or the range of jobs available.[3] The potential of career changers was perhaps most readily seen in the approaches adopted to recruit the mass vaccination workforce in 2021. Of the 2,000 people recruited to six mass vaccination centres in West London from the unemployed or people who had been furloughed, 40% stated that they wished to continue working in the NHS when the centres were wound down. Over half were from BAME communities.[4]

BOX 3.8 NATIONAL CAREERS SERVICE (NCS)

The NCS is a government supported service that provides people in England, aged 13 years old or above, with careers information, advice and guidance. Assistance is also given to schools and others who assist people to make career choices. Services provided include helping people, of whatever age, explore career options, skills assessment to support career choices (when I completed the NCS careers survey it suggested a future as a museum attendant, a community development manager and publican – none of which frankly are unappealing) and information about education and training people might need to pursue their chosen careers.

Structural changes in the labour market, such as increased automation, may lead to more people seeking to change carers (Deloitte Insights, 2018). Analyse by the ONS (2019) found that jobs with word such as 'patient' and 'care' in their job descriptions were at low risk of automation. Many support workers, as we have seen, are in fact career changers, having worked in other sectors, particularly retail and hospitality, before joining the NHS. Fully optimising the potential of career changers, though, requires national programmes, such as the HEE AHP one, including media campaigns; however, engagement with employment partners locally, particularly council economic teams and NCS, can facilitate transition in localities.

Supporting people into NHS jobs

Some people experience barriers to employment. This may be because they have been unemployed for some time, or have a disability, a criminal record, have recently left the care system, they may have a significant health condition, or are recovering from drug and alcohol misuse or are a refugee. Barriers can include negative stereotyping. For people with disabilities this may mean an inaccurate belief that as employees they will have poor attendance and a limited ability to perform (Griffin, 2022). Associated with this is also a lack of understanding about the benefits such individuals can bring to organisations – which are in fact considerable. Particular barriers exist when individuals require adjustments to be made, including to recruitment processes. Young people leaving the care system, for instance may not have had many opportunities to gain work experience. A stress on prior experience in job advertisements would clearly disadvantage them. People with a learning disability may require an Easy Read application form.

Outside/In GYO approaches to workforce planning actively seek to support people who experience obstacles to employment – and for good reason. Supporting people who are disadvantaged in the labour market not only builds workplace capacity, particularly as such individuals are likely to have low quit rates once employed, as well as demonstrating an employer's commitment to equality and diversity but also because employment is a significant social determinant of health and wellbeing helps reduce health inequalities (Health Foundation, 2018; Kessler et al., 2021). Other benefits accruing from support employment include increased job satisfaction for existing staff, improved organisational productivity, better staff morale and reduced staff turnover (Beyer and Beyer, 2017). In a review of the peer reviewed literature Griffin (2022) found the following benefits that research had identified when people with disabilities secured paid employment:

- Financial independence.
- Improved sense of belonging.
- Improved health and wellbeing.
- Increased self-efficacy.
- Reduced social isolation and greater participation in society.

One barrier that some people can face is that many employers, including in the NHS, believe that supported employment requires significant resources, such as physical adjustments to working environments. Whilst some employees may require additional support, resources are often available to assist transition into work. Support is available, for example, through the *Access to Work* scheme for people with a disability or health condition and their employers, to enable adjustments or adaptions in the workplace (such as the provision of special equipment) as well as help getting to and from work. Mental health support is also provided, where necessary. Mencap (n.d.) found that the average adjustment cost for organisations was just £75.30 and for over half (55%) of employers this was a one-off cost. Any cost incurred need to be seen alongside the benefits of recruiting staff who are, in the case of people with disabilities, 3.5 times more likely to stay in their jobs than their non-disabled colleagues (ibid.).

BOX 3.9 WHAT IS SUPPORTED EMPLOYMENT?

Supported employment is a term that has been used to describe a personalised model of employment support that aims to assist people who may need help into work and to support them once employed to retain employment. Although initially used to describe approaches to support people with disabilities, it can apply to any individual requiring assistance. Behind the model is a belief that anyone can be employed, and retain work, if sufficient support is provided. A principle of support employment is that people gain the training they need to work once employed, rather than having acquired it before. Individuals are supported through tailor-made assistance designed to not only help them retain employment but also to progress their careers (British Association for Supported Employment, n.d.).

Delivering effective supported employment programmes involves collaborative working. Specialist and approved employment support agencies, such as The Princes Trust, work with disadvantaged individuals to identify their aspirations, experience, skill and learning needs. Colleges may provide work-ready training. Local authorities will also have an interest. Employment of young people with Special Education Needs and Disabilities will require working with education settings.

Supporting young people with disabilities into NHS employment

People with learning disabilities, autism, physical and/or sensory impairments can be particularly disadvantaged in the workplace, experiencing rates of unemployment twice as high as people without disabilities (Kessler et al., 2021). People with disabilities are also, compared with the population as a whole, significantly more likely to be underemployed, experience high levels of job insecurity and lower hourly earnings. In 2019, 53.2% of people with a disability were employed. For people with a severe learning disability this rate fell to just 17.6% – the lowest rate of any disability (ONS, 2019). People with disabilities are also more likely to suffer during economic downturns in terms of losing their jobs or cuts in pay (Jones et al., 2021). *The NHS Long Term Plan* (NHS England, 2019a) committed the NHS to increasing the number of supported employment opportunities it provided for people with disabilities and to deliver employment outcomes for at least half of those on programmes, an aspiration reinforced in the *NHS Interim People Plan* (NHS England, 2019b). In 2021, however, just 30 trusts provide a supported employment opportunity, less than an eighth of the total (Kessler et al., 2021).

Most supported employment opportunities that are provided by the NHS are for young people (those aged under 25 years) age, with a Special Education Need or Disability (SEND). young people assessed by their local authority as having significant needs requiring additional support are provided with an *Education and Health Care Plan* (EHCP). EHCPs include objectives to assist the individual to transition into adulthood and paid work. EHCPs remain in place until someone reaches 25 years of age. If not employed, young people with SEND attend mainstream schools, special schools or colleges.

There are a number of supported employment programmes for young people with SEND in the NHS operated by agencies such as The Princes Trust, Mencap, Project Choice or DFN Project Search (see Box 3.10 below). Many of these focus on supported internships, which are structured programmes delivered in partnership with education settings, typically lasting a year, that include a period of work experience as well as formal teaching of employment and job-related skills. Supported internships have been shown to produce better outcomes for young people with autism and learning disabilities, in terms of sustained employment and wage levels, compared to young people who have not accessed such schemes (Timmons et al., 2012).

BOX 3.10 PARTNERSHIPS AND PATHWAYS: THE NORTH WEST LONDON SEND SUPPORTED EMPLOYMENT STRATEGY

Since 2018 NHS trusts, local authorities, the North West London ICS and other partners have worked together to increase the number of opportunities for local young people with SEND. In 2021 increasing employment rates for young people with disabilities became a formal objective in the ICS's population health strategy – underlining the role support employment can play in reducing health inequalities. The system-wide supported employment strategy comprises the following features:

1. It is 'end to end' starting with careers information, advice and guidance linked to work experience, traineeships, internships, volunteering, appropriate recruitment and retention, employment support and ending with career progression and development, including apprenticeships.
2. It is 'joined-up' with other relevant strategies including aligning with the West London council's economic strategy.
3. It is system-based with employers, and other partners, working together to deliver programmes, share expertise, insights and resources.

The programme has been led by Amanda Griffiths whose post, although based in Ealing Council is funded by the ICS in a systems integrator role across the area. She told me that from 'an employment rate of 5.6% for this cohort partnerships with local trusts are consistently achieving 60% plus employment rates. The model is based on partnership working across the system to raise expectations and skills for employment starting with schools and focusing on those with significant learning needs. The programme raises awareness and preparation for employment with students, families, and education providers and employer stakeholders coordinated regionally with a SEND specialist who has a joint role across the WLA and the NHS bringing together the stakeholders at each stage of the pathway and supporting stakeholders to establish provision' (interview with author). Seven of the eight NHS trusts in the ICS footprint in 2022 either had supported employment programmes or were planning to introduce them.

The NHS Learning Disability Employment Programme

The NHS Learning Disability Employment Programme (LDEP) was established to provide NHS employers with resources to increase recruitment of people with a learning disability or autism. LDEP's overall aim is for the NHS to lead the way as an employer of disabled people. *The NHS Long Term Plan* (NHS England, 2019a) set a clear commitment for the NHS to employ more people with autism or a learning disability. A central element of the LDEP is an employer three-step 'Pledge', which commits NHS organisations (providers, commissioners and arm's-length bodies) to deliver tangible outcomes in respect of supported employment. Step 1 requires organisation commitment to supported employment. Step 2 requires planning to introduce programmes and Step 3 introducing those programmes. Launched in 2015 by 2021 more than 120 organisations had signed the pledge.

Disability Confident Employer

NHS employers signing the LDEP Pledge are required to obtain accreditation as a *Disability Confident Employer.* This is an official government scheme that seeks to ensure organisations have accessible application processes so that disabled people are able to apply for jobs and once employed adjustments are made to support them in work. Support is available from local Job Centre Plus offices to assist employers. There are three levels to the scheme. The LDEP Pledge requires NHS employers to at least meet the second level. Organisations, self-assess their recruitment strategies, in-work support and development opportunities for people with disabilities.

The Work and Health Programme

The Work and Health Programme is voluntary for people who have been unemployed for up 24 months (and compulsory for those who have been out of work for longer than that). The aim of the scheme is to assist people to find and prepare for work. Support available for individuals includes identifying their employment needs, matching their skills to available work, acting as an interface with employers, providing training and helping manage any health problems that might impact on work.

In addition, people with disabilities who are older than 25 years of age can also be supported via *The Work and Health Programme*, through an *Intensive Personalised Employment Scheme* which provides one-to-one assistance to adults with a disability and/or a health condition. This normally lasts for 15 months but can include a further six months support for those in employment.

There are also employment programmes supported by government, local authorities, charities and the voluntary sector organisations that seek to target support for specific groups, such as looked after children, people in prisons or the probation service, for example. Whilst delivered by different agencies in different parts of the country, most (and particularly those commissioned to provide *The Health and Work Programme*) will be known or overseen by local authorities again showing the importance of engaging with local employment and skills systems.

How to make supported employment a success

Whilst the benefits of delivering supported employment schemes should be clear, there are challenges that need to be addressed in designing and sustaining such schemes. In his review of supported employment schemes for young people with SEND in West London, Griffin (2022) found those involved in the programmes (see Box 3.10) reported the following issues that they had to address:

- Matching supply with demand. One trust that had wanted to run a scheme for SEND young people, but a suitable cohort was not available in their locality. Close working with council SEND leads will help ensure recruits are available.
- Stereotyping. There was a view that certain services or support roles were not suitable for the young people with SEND. Risk assessments were undertaken before any placement and it was discovered that young people's interests and skills could be matched with a wide range of opportunities as Box 3.11 below illustrates, including patient facing ones. Working as a system allowed stereotypes to be challenged because employers were able to learn from each other.
- Capacity. Engaging with services, planning placements, liaising with external stakeholders, managing cohorts and dealing with day-to-day issues required additional capacity. Some of this was met from external partners including the local council, some had to be found by NHS trusts internally. The support of senior leadership including trust boards was crucial here as was a recognition that over time there was a return on investment (through reduced vacancy rates).
- Not every person on the programmed was 'work ready'. One council lead pointed out that some people on supported employment programmes 'may have been unemployed for ten or fifteen years' (p. 12). One solution to this,

adopted by the area, was to offer a range of programmes including traineeships, tailored to individual need.

• Participants identified the need to integrate and join up supported employment with wider workforce strategies, noted 'supported internships can be a ghetto'

What, though, are the approaches that help make supported employment programmes a success? Much of the evidence summarised below, could in fact apply to Outside/In GYO workforce approaches more generally. Research (Kessler et al., 2021; Griffin, 2022) suggests there is a need to:

• Make appropriate adjustments to existing HR processes, for example ensuring it is clear in job advertisements that the organisation actively values diversity and inclusion along with the use of Easy Ready job descriptions and application forms.
• The development of inclusive workplace cultures that truly value diversity. Leadership has a key role to play in shifting cultures. Understanding the benefits of supported employment contributes and awareness training for existing staff.
• Supportive management.
• The deployment of 'Buddies' and 'Mentors' to assist those being supported into work.
• The integration of those on the supported employment programme into the teams.
• The identification of suitable posts that could be filled.
• An end-to-end approach that starts with careers information and continues to employment and progression.

BOX 3.11 WHAT ROLES CAN PEOPLE WITH DISABILITIES DO IN THE NHS?

There are a vast number of jobs that people with disabilities can undertake – with the right support and training, including (Griffin, 2022):

Healthcare Assistant
Endoscopy Assistant
Radiology Assistant
Laboratory Support
Warehouse Operative
Print Room Operative
Human Resource Support
Maintenance Restaurant Assistant

Retail
Library Support
Administrative Support Worker
Leaning and Knowledge Assistant
Payroll Administrator
Receptionist
Finance Administrator
Recruitment Administration Support
Call Centre Support
Theatre Health Care Assistant
Domestic Operative
Ward Host
Back of House Operative
Porter
Post Room Assistant
Storeroom Assistant Health Records
Waste Management
Laundry Assistant
Ward Reception

Conclusion

This has been a long section, reflecting the complex infrastructure that surrounds the recruitment and employment of people with disabilities as well as other groups that experience barriers when seeking work. Working together with external partners and accessing the resources and support available, whether from Job Centre Plus or council employment teams or specialist employment support agencies, is key to delivering successful supported employment programmes in the NHS. Doing so will not only help address workforce shortages but also improve workforce diversity, performance as well as contributing to population health. Getting this right from the start will lay the foundations for an inclusive workplace culture that allows people to not only remain working in the NHS but progress their careers.

I played only a small part in the North West London supported employment strategy (see Box 3.10). In 2017 I sat in the lecture theatre in Charing Cross Hospital at a graduation ceremony for a cohort of DFN Project Search interns who had successfully completed their internships in the hospital. Next to me sat a parent. He was in tears. When I asked if he was ok, he told me that he had never imagined that his son, who had autism, would ever be able to work, and now, thanks to the NHS trust and its partners, his son had a job which gave him independence and boosted his confidence. This moment bought home to me more than anything the importance of supported employment.

Volunteering, traineeships, work experience and job shadowing

We have seen that there are a number of labour supply routes that the NHS could use for recruitment into support worker vacancies, along with the importance of raising awareness of NHS careers and working with labour market partners, particularly schools, colleges and local authorities. Research suggests that interventions that provide people with direct experience of a career can be particularly effective in engaging them (Mann et al., 2014; Education and Employers Research, 2018a). There are a number of ways that people can get a 'taste' of NHS employment: volunteering, traineeships, job shadowing and work experience. These are all integral elements of Outside/In GYO and need to be deployed as part of a deliberate and joined up strategy.

Volunteers

Volunteers have long been a feature of healthcare services but *The NHS Long Term Plan* (NHS England 2019a) committed to invest £2.3 million to support a growth in the number of volunteers from 78,000 in 2020 to 156,000 in 2024. Volunteers can be found across the NHS, including in primary care, and perform a very wide range of roles that include being a trustee, a hospital radio DJ, navigators, interpreters, fundraisers, providing peer support and acting as advocates (Pro Bono Economics, n.d.; NHS England, 2017).

Volunteers play an important role helping to improve the service user experience, as well as building stronger links between services and communities, supporting integration and improving public health and reducing health inequalities (Naylor et al., 2013).

NHS staff recognise the value of volunteers, although there may be concerns that they will be used to replace paid staff (Ross et al., 2018). As a result employers do need to consider how volunteers are deployed by developing a volunteer strategy. This means ensuring clear boundaries between volunteers and employed staff through job descriptions, induction and on-going training. In addition, training should be provided to employees to raise their awareness of volunteers and improve their interaction with them (Rose et al., 2018).

BOX 3.12 HELPFORCE VOLUNTEER CHARTER

Developed with NHS trade unions and professional bodies, Helpforce, an organisation that seeks to increase volunteering opportunities in the NHS, developed a volunteers' charter based on the following principles (Helpforce, n.d.):

1. Volunteers will not undermine current or future paid roles in the health workforce, and tasks to meet the essential health and care needs of patients and service users will always be undertaken by paid staff.

2. Volunteers will never be included in any counts of staffing levels and will wear uniforms/badges that clearly distinguish them from staff.
3. NHS trade unions should be engaged at local level in setting out and monitoring the way that volunteers are deployed within the organisation, with the need to maintain patient safety and confidentiality as the key consideration.

For the purpose of Outside/In GYO workforce strategies volunteering is an opportunity for a wide range of people, including those with disabilities, to experience healthcare and as a potential pool of recruits.

Traineeships

Traineeships are programmes aimed at helping people transition into work, either immediately or in the future. They combine experience of work, education and acquisition of employability skills. Common in many countries (for an assessment of the policy in Italy see Cappellini et al., 2019 for instance) they were originally launched in Britain as a national programme by the Coalition government in 2013. This traineeship scheme was open to young people aged 19–24 years old, without the necessary skills or experience to enter work and/or an apprenticeship; a gap the scheme sought to meet.

Although mentioned in passing in *Talent for Care* (HEE, 2014), traineeships do not appear to have become widespread in the NHS. Indeed traineeships generally declined in Britain, from a peak of 24,100 starts in 2015/16, to around 14,000 in 2019/20 (*FE Week*, n.d.) In 2020, however, the government relaunched them and set a target to grow the number of starts to 40,000. This was supported by an investment of £111 million to assist employers who took a trainee on (Employment and Skills Funding Agency, 2020). The new traineeship scheme has the following features:

- It is open to 19–24 year olds (or 25 years old if the young person has an *ECHP*).
- Trainees can possess a qualification up to RQF level 3.
- Traineeships can last for a minimum of 6 weeks and for a maximum of a year.
- They include a work placement lasting at least 70 hours.
- Trainees receive preparation for work training, including on CV writing.
- Trainees receive assistance with English and Mathematics attainment and digital skills.
- Trainees are not guaranteed pay or expenses.

As before, the aim of the scheme is to provide young people with work related skills in preparation for employment. Evidence suggests from this perspective traineeships are effective. After twelve months of completing a traineeship, 75% of trainees either commenced employment or went on to further study (FE Week, n.d.)

Traineeships provide the NHS with another means of providing support to young people into employment.

Work experience

Work experience refers to time spent in a workplace learning about a job, organisation and career. Often thought of in terms of younger people, work experience should also be considered for adults, particularly potential career changers. Exposure to healthcare settings, workplaces and occupations can play a significant role influencing career choices (Sok et al., 2017). Other benefits accruing from running work experience programmes for participants include (HEE, 2014):

• Helping to raise ambitions.
• Providing insights into the reality of work.
• Developing employment skills.
• Challenging stereotypes.

Work experience can be for a short duration or longer term, structured or informal, in a clinical or non-clinical settings, in person or virtual. In 2014 HEE undertook a survey of NHS trusts and found that work experience opportunities were provided by all NHS trusts, but that the actual numbers available varied from 100 a year to 800 (ibid.). The survey also found that the most common way they were arranged was through individual or family connections. This meant in the words of HEE that work experience could be 'a lottery' and 'that opportunities are most likely to be taken by those with social networks and links' often people wishing to assist their application to a healthcare degree (ibid., 30).

The HEE (ibid.) findings suggest a lack of work experience strategies in the NHS. As with all Outside/In GYO approaches to workforce supply there is a need to join work experience up with other interventions and ensure opportunities are fairly accessible, particularly for groups that may be underrepresented in the workforce. Working with schools and colleges, for example, could create the opportunity for young people interested in studying a health-related T Levels to gain some experience before they start or even formally apply. Supported employment strategies should also include work experience as an element. More practically the organisation of work experience requires consideration of: capacity for placements, the development of resources such as information about the organisation, and clarity about who is responsible for the programmes, HEE (2014b) found that this was most often the trust's Learning and Development lead or secondly HR. Finally, the effectiveness of placements should be regularly reviewed and assessed.

Job shadowing

Job (or work) shadowing allows perspective NHS employees to directly observe a healthcare professional carrying out their work normally for up to a week. It is an opportunity to not only find out about a role, but also how the NHS operates and ask questions. Whilst focused on shadowing registered staff (particularly medics) there is an opportunity, as with work experience, to give people, including career changes, experience of support roles, as well as providing support workers with developmental opportunities. Again, as with work experience systems can come together to develop ICS-wide job shadowing strategies and ensure that schools and colleges in less affluent areas are engaged.

Conclusion: Building bridges to grow your own workforce

This chapter has discussed the role of the NHS as an anchor institution in its local community and the important part it has to play, particularly as an employer, contributing to social value and improving population health. The factors that shape people's decisions (or not) to work in healthcare have also been considered along the interventions, including the role of NHS Ambassadors, that can assist awareness raising including of support worker careers and the wide range of occupations within the NHS. Securing the workforce of the future is a vital task the NHS faces, and we have looked at sources of labour that have traditionally been underutilised such as college students and people who experience barriers to employment. Volunteering, work experience, job shadowing and traineeships provide people with an opportunity to experience the realities of working in the NHS. All these are part of an Outside/In GYO approach to workforce planning.

Outside/In GYO approaches are not just about *what* happens; they are also about *who* delivers the interventions – the fact they are based on collaboration with partners, such as Job Centre Plus, in local employment and skill systems. The Future College Commission report with the NHS Confederation (2020) reported that the NHS found the college sector 'hard to navigate' (p. 10). On the college's side it was felt that 'the complexity of the NHS can make it difficult for training and education partners to fully understand and engage in the right discussions about health and care system development at the right time' (ibid., 11).

ICSs create the opportunity to address this complexity through system-wide collaboration. ICSs also create the opportunity for single points of contact to allow partners such as schools, community groups and colleges to connect, particularly if 'navigator' roles have been created (ibid.). ICSs can also assist delivery of economies of scale when developing and delivering Outside/In GYO workforce interventions.

The NHS has long experienced staff shortages, and high turnover particularly for support worker roles. There are large numbers of people who would like to work for the NHS. Some of them are at school, some are in colleges, some are unemployed, some work in other occupations, some are receiving benefits, some may not even know that they would like to work in the NHS yet because they are not aware of the wide range of careers available. Some may be confused whether they have the right knowledge, skills or values. An analogy for this might be a V-shaped valley. On one side are people looking for jobs, on the other the NHS that needs people to work for it. The Outside/In GYO strategies described in this chapter can bridge the gap. To do so may require the creation of navigator roles that act as go-betweens bringing partners together with minimum disruption to their day-to-day jobs, helping to build lasting relations. Working with local partners such as colleges and local authorities will not only be cost effective, but also deliver wider benefits including lower turnover and a workforce that better reflects its local population.

Checklist

Engagement with local employment systems can occur at individual employer level, including PCNs, as well as systems-level and regionally (for example across a devolved authority). In developing Outside/In GYO workforce strategies and planning to engage with local partners, there are a number of points for the NHS to consider (HEE, 2021):

- What links are already in place there with local labour and skill system organisations, particularly colleges and local authorities? Where are there gaps?
- Is the NHS engaged with local economic strategies including membership of relevant groups?
- Are NHS employers/systems able to articulate their employment and skills needs to providers?
- Have single points of contact been established for external partners?
- Do employer, system or regional workforce plans include GYO targets and interventions?
- Are GYO approaches aligned with health objectives, for example the need to address health inequalities or promote public health?
- Is the composition of the workforce – at all levels – known? Has this been mapped against the diversity of local communities? To what extent are support workers recruited from local labour markets (for example directly following school or college education)?
- Are senior leaders within organisations committed to Outside/In GYO approaches?
- Is there clear responsibility within organisations for Outside/In GYO interventions?
- Does the organisation/system have a formal strategy for schools and college engagement and associated resources (including ICS-wide strategies)? This strategy could include identifying particular NHS careers that employers wish to promote and collectively recruiting, training and supporting NHS Ambassadors? The degree to which the NHS engages with local schools and colleges should be assessed particularly to ensure those education settings in less affluent areas are included.
- What form does engagement take? What activities are not undertaken that could be?
- Does engagement start with primary schools?

- Are links made with National Careers Service so that their advisors for example are aware of the full range of NHS jobs?
- Are supported employment opportunities provided for adults and young people who may experience barriers to work?
- Are supported employment opportunities 'end-to-end', meaning that they begin with careers information, embrace recruitment and selection processes, includes traineeships, work experience, job shadowing and volunteering, as well as in-work support?
- Is there an organisational/system structured approach to work experience, volunteering, job shadowing and traineeships, that (1) includes support worker roles, (2) is inclusive (i.e., ensures access regardless of background) and (3) is linked to Outside/In GYO targets such as increasing the amount of local people employed by the NHS?

Notes

1 A report in 2020 found that rugby league clubs generated an additional £185 million in social value in their local communities (www.nwemail.co.uk/sport/19003069.rugby-lea gue-clubs-social-impact-worth-185-million/).
2 Authors interview with National Careers Service (London) and research conducted by the Vice Chair of Association of Business Psychologists in 2019 (unpublished).
3 Source: discussion with author.
4 Unpublished survey by the North West London ICS.

References

Asaria, M., Doran, T. and Cookson, R. (2016). The costs of inequality: Whole-population modelling study of lifetime inpatient hospital costs in the English National Health Service by level of neighbourhood deprivation. *Journal of Epidemiology and Community Health*. https://jech.bmj.com/content/70/10/990

Association of Colleges (2020). *College Key Facts 2019/2020*. Available from: www.aoc.co.uk/sites/default/files/AoC%20College%20Key%20Facts%202019-20.pdf

Augar, P. (2019). *Independent Panel Report to the Post-18 Review of Education and Funding*. Department of Education. Available from: https://assets.publishing.service.gov.uk/gov ernment/uploads/system/uploads/attachment_data/file/805127/Review_of_post_18_ education_and_funding.pdf

Beyer, S. and Beyer, A. (2017) *A Systematic Review of the Benefits for Employers of Employing People with Learning Disabilities*. London: Mencap. Available from: www.mencap.org. uk/sites/default/files/2017-06/2017.061%20Benefits%20of%20employing%20P WLD%255b1%255d%20%281%29.pdf

British Association for Supported Employment (n.d.). *What Is Supported Employment?* British Association for Supported Employment. Available from: www.base-uk.org/what-suppor ted-employment

Cappenllini, E., Maitino, M., Patacchini, V. and Sciclone, N. (2019). Are traineeships stepping-stones for youth working careers in Italy? *International Journal of Manpower*, 40(8), 1389–1410. https://doi.org/10.1108/IJM-03-2018-0099

CBI/Pearsons (2019). *Education and Learning for the Modern World: CBI/Pearsons Education and Skills Survey Results 2019.* Available from: www.cbi.org.uk/media/3841/12546_te ss_2019.pdf

The Centre for Local Economic Strategies (2016). *Skills Policy that Works for All.* The Centre for Local Economic Strategies. Available from: https://cles.org.uk/wp-content/uploads/2016/10/Skills-policy-that-works-for-all1.pdf

The Centre for Local Economic Strategies (2021). *What Is an Anchor Institution?* The Centre for Local Economic Strategies. https://cles.org.uk/what-is-community-wealth-build ing/what-is-an-anchor-institution/

Deloitte Insights (2018). *Redefine Work. The Untapped Opportunity of Expanding Value.* Available from: www2.deloitte.com/content/dam/insights/us/articles/4779_Redefine-work/DI_Redefine-work.pdf

Department for Education (2019). *Teacher Recruitment and Retention Strategy.* Available from: www.gov.uk/government/publications/teacher-recruitment-and-retention-strategy

De Smet, A., Dowling, B., Mugayer-Baldocchi, M. and Schaniger, B. (2021). Great attrition or great attraction? The choice is yours. *Mckinsey Quarterly*, 8 September 2021. Available from: www.mckinsey.com/business-functions/organization/our-insights/great-attrition-or-great-attraction-the-choice-is-yours).

Education and Employers and HEE (2021). *NHS Ambassadors: How You've Helped 400,000 Young People.* Available from: www.hee.nhs.uk/sites/default/files/documents/NHS%20 Ambassadors%20Impact%20Report%20-%20June%202021%20%28FINAL%29.pdf

Edwards, N. (n.d). *NHS Buildings: Obstacles or Opportunities.* Kings Fund. www.kingsfund.org.uk/sites/default/files/field/field_publication_file/perspectives-estates-nhs-property-nigel-edwards-jul13.pdf

Employers and Education (2018a) *Employer Engagement in Education: Insights from International Evidence for Effective Practice and Future Research.* Education Endowment Foundation. Available from: www.educationandemployers.org/research/employerengagementined ucation/

Employers and Education. (2018b). *Envisioning the Future of Education and Jobs – Trends, Data and Drawings.* Available from: www.educationandemployers.org/research/oecd-joint-report/

Employment and Skills Funding Agency (2020). *Traineeship Information for Trainees.* Available from: www.gov.uk/guidance/traineeship-information-for-trainees

FE Week (n.d.). *The Revival of Traineeships.* Available from: https://feweek.co.uk/wp-content/uploads/2020/10/traineeships-supp-2020-A4-digi-update.pdf

Glerean, N., Hupil, M., Talman, K. and Haavisto, E. (2017). Young peoples' perceptions of the nursing profession: An integrative review. *Nurse Education Today* 57, 95–102. https://doi.org/10.1016/j.nedt.2017.07.008

Griffin, R. (2022). *Making Change Happen. Working as a System to Increase Supported Employment. A Report to NHS England and London Councils.* (Forthcoming).

Health Foundation (2018). Building Healthier Communities: The role of the NHS as an anchor institution. Available from: www.health.org.uk/publications/reports/building-healthier-communities-role-of-nhs-as-anchor-institution

Health Foundation (2021a). Unequal pandemic, Fairer recovery. Available from: www.health.org.uk/publications/reports/unequal-pandemic-fairer-recovery

Health Foundation (2021b). Lifelong learning and levelling up: building blocks for good health. Why further education is critical to the levelling up agenda. Available from: www.health.org.uk/publications/long-reads/lifelong-learning-and-levelling-up-building-blo cks-for-good-health

HEE (2014a). *Talent for Care. A National Strategic Framework to Develop the Healthcare Support Workforce.* Available from: www.hee.nhs.uk/sites/default/files/documents/TfC%20Natio nal%20Strategic%20Framework_0.pdf

HEE (2014b). *Widening Participation It Matters. Our Strategy and Initial Action Plan.* Available from: www.hee.nhs.uk/sites/default/files/documents/Widening%20Participation%20it%20Matters_0.pdf

HEE (2021) *AHP Support Workforce – Grow Your Own Workforce strategies.* www.hee.nhs.uk/sites/default/files/documents/ahp_guide_gyo_acc.pdf

HEE (2022). Career change to AHP. Webpage. Available from: (www.hee.nhs.uk/our-work/allied-health-professions/stimulate-demand/career-change-ahp)

HEE (n.d.). *What Comes Next? National Strategic Framework for Engagement with Schools and Communities to Build a Diverse Healthcare Workforce.* Available from: www.hee.nhs.uk/sites/default/files/documents/Strategic%20Framework%20-%20What%20Comes%20Next.pdf

Helpforce (n.d.). *Charter to Strengthen Relations between the Helpforce Programme and Staff in the National Health Service England.* Helpforce. Available from: https://storage.googleapis.com/helpforce/publications/Helpforce-Unison-Charter.pdf?mtime=20200225093335&focal=none

Institute of Government. (2020). NHS Procurement. Web page. Available from: www.instituteforgovernment.org.uk/explainers/nhs-procurement

Jones, M., Hoque, K. Wass, V. and Bacon, N. (2021). Inequality and the economic cycle: Disabled employees' experience of work during the Great Recession in Britain. *British Journal of Industrial Relations* 58(3), 788–815. 10.1111/bjir.12577

Kessler, I., Griffin, R. and Griffiths, A. (2021). *Supported Employment Programme in NHS Trusts for Young People with Disabilities: Piecing the Puzzle Together.* London, King's College London. Available from: www.hee.nhs.uk/printpdf/our-work/talent-care-widening-participation/supported-employment-programme-nhs-trusts-young-people-disabilities-piecing-puzzle-together

Kluczynska, U. (2016). Motives for choosing and resigning from nursing by men and the definition of masculinity: a qualitative study. *Journal of Advanced Nursing* 73(6), 1366–1376. https://doi.org/10.1111/jan.13240

Learning Disability Employment Programme (2022) NHS Learning Disability Employment Programme. Increasing the number of people with a learning disability and/or autism employed in the NHS. Webpage. Available from: www.england.nhs.uk/about/equality/equality-hub/ld-emp-prog/

Leavey, C., Bunbury, S. and Cresswell, R. (2021). *Lifelong Learning and Levelling Up: Building Blocks for Good Health. Why Further Education is Critical to the Levelling Up Agenda.* Health Foundation. Available from: www.health.org.uk/publications/long-reads/lifelong-learning-and-levelling-up-building-blocks-for-good-health

Mann, A. and Dawkins, J. (2014) Employer engagement in education: Literature review. *Education and Employers.* Available from: www.educationandemployers.org/research/employer-engagement-in-education-literature-review-janaury-2014/

Meacham, H., Cavanaugh, J., Shaw, A. and Bartram, T. (2017). HRM practices that support the employment and social inclusion of workers with an intellectual disability, *Personnel Review* 46(8), 1475–1492.

Mencap (n.d.). *Good for Business. The Benefits of Employing People with a Learning Disability.* Available from: www.mencap.org.uk/sites/default/files/2017-06/2017.080.1%20LDW%202017%20guide%20DIGITAL%20V2.pdf

Naylor, C., Mundle, C., Weaks, L. and Buck, D. (2013). *Volunteering in Health and Care. Securing a Sustainable Future.* The Kings Fund, available from: www.kingsfund.org.uk/sites/default/files/field/field_publication_file/volunteering-in-health-and-social-care-kingsfund-mar13.pdf

NHS Confederation and The College of the Future (2020). *Creating the Workforce of the Future: A New Collaborative Approach for the NHS and Colleges in England.* Available from: www.nhsconfed.org/sites/default/files/media/Creating-the-workforce-of-the-future_4.pdf

NHS England (2017). *Recruiting and Managing Volunteers in NHS Providers. A Practical Guide.* Available from: www.england.nhs.uk/wp-content/uploads/2017/10/recruiting-manag ing-volunteers-nhs-providers-practical-guide.pdf

NHS England (2019). *The NHS Long Term Plan.* Available from: www.longtermplan.nhs.uk

Office of National Statistics (2019). *Disability and Employment UK: 2019.* Available from: www.ons.gov.uk/peoplepopulationandcommunity/healthandsocialcare/disability/ bulletins/disabilityandemploymentuk/2019

Parker, K. (2021). Williamson: My vision for T levels to be international. TES, 27 April 2021. Available from: www.tes.com/magazine/archived/williamson-my-vision-t-levels-be- international

Pro Bono Economics (n.d.). *Could Skilled Volunteering Help Transform the NHS?* Available from: https://storage.googleapis.com/helpforce/publications/Skilled-Volunteering-Rep ort-1.pdf?mtime=20200225093338&focal=none

Rogers, M., Chambers, N. and Percy, C. (2020). *Disconnected: Career Aspirations and Jobs in the UK.* Education and Employers. Available from: www.educationandemployers.org/wp- content/uploads/2020/01/Disconnected-Career-aspirations-and-jobs-in-the-UK-1.pdf

Ross, S., Fenney, D., Ward, D. and Buck, D. (2018) *The Role of Volunteers in the NHS. Views from the Frontline.* The Kings Fund. Available from: www.kingsfund.org.uk/sites/default/ files/2018-12/Role_volunteers_NHS_December_2018.pdf

Sok, Y. K. L., Ling, T. W., Yeow, L. C., Siriwan, L. and Khoon, K. T. (2017). Career choice and perceptions of nursing amongst healthcare students in higher education intuitions. *Nurse Education Today* 52, 66–72.

TenHove, Y., Castelein, S., Jansen, G. and Roodbol, P., (2017). Dreams and disappointments regarding nursing: Student nurses' reasons for attrition and retention. A qualitative study design. *Nurse Education Today* 54, 28–36.

Vosper, M. R., Price, R. C. and Ashmore, L. A. (2005). Careers and destinations of radiog- raphy students from the University of Hertfordshire. *Radiography* 11, 79–88.

Widdowson, J. and King, M. (n.d.). *Higher Education in Further Education: Leading the Challenge.* Further Education Trust for Leadership. Available from: https://fetl.org.uk/publications/ higher-education-in-further-education-leading-the-challenge/

Williams, J. (2013). *Constructing New Professional Identities: Career Changers in Teacher Education.* Sense Publishers, Rotterdam.

Wu, L. T., Low, M. M. J., Tan, K. K., Lopez, V. and Law, S. Y. (2015). Why not nursing? A system- atic review of factors influencing career choice amongst healthcare students. *International Nursing Review* 58, 547–562.

PART II
Get in

4

ON-BOARDING

Recruitment, selection, induction and initial training of support workers

Introduction

In the last chapter we considered how to raise awareness of NHS careers, including support worker ones, and how to attract and, in some cases support, people to work in healthcare jobs. This chapter is concerned with on-boarding – the 'Get In' stage of the career cycle and the second element that constitutes Outside/In GYO workforce strategies. On-boarding encompasses recruitment and selection, induction and approximately the first year of employment. For support workers this is the time they complete *The Care Certificate*.

This chapter reviews approaches to recruitment and selection, including new models that are being developed in some parts of the country, value-based recruitment, induction and *The Care Certificate* including the *Accelerated Care Certificate* process developed during Covid-19.

The importance of getting on-boarding right

Starting a new job for anyone can be a confusing and anxious time, as well as an exciting experience. Getting on-boarding right is important because the initial weeks and months of employment are critical as new staff orientate and socialise themselves to their job, team and organisations. However, if the on-boarding experience is not well organised or does not meet new staff's expectations, ultimately, they may leave. The contribution, for good or ill, on-boarding makes to turnover is illustrated by the fact that 42% of companies surveyed by the Chartered Institute for Personnel and Development (CIPD) in 2020, reported that they planned to improve their induction processes.

The nature of healthcare work means that a new starter's early experience of NHS employment is perhaps even more critical than in many other organisations.

DOI: 10.4324/9781003251620-9

There is a body of evidence investigating what is described as the 'transition shock' healthcare degree students, such as newly qualified nurses, can face when starting employment after graduating. For newly qualified graduates, a literature review by HEE (n.d.) found that stress and 'burnout [is] particularly high … turnover rates tend to be high in the first year of qualification and remain high, or even rise during the second year of service before declining' (p. 2). This stress and burnout derive from newly qualified staff experiencing the realities of a care job; not just the various aspects of patient care, but also working practices such as long shifts and weekend working (see Wakefield, 2018, for example and Box 4.2 below). One study estimated that 34% of newly qualified nurses do not go on to register to practice (Finlayson et al., 2002). Drawing again from the research literature on newly qualified nurses, HEE's (n.d.) review of the evidence found that where there was high turnover amongst new recruits this contributed to a feeling amongst those that remained that they were 'survivors' (p. 9).

BOX 4.1 *THE HEALTHCARE SUPPORT WORKER (HCSW) 2020 CAMPAIGN*

On 9 September 2020, the Chief Nursing Officer for England, Ruth May, launched a national nursing support worker recruitment campaign called *Healthcare Support Worker 2020 (HCSW2020)* to support NHS trusts recruit people into nursing support worker roles. Reducing support worker vacancies were seen as a means of reducing reliance on temporary staffing, of improving continuity of care, creating a progression route into registered posts, as well as increasing support worker capacity in line with aspirations of *The NHS Long Term Plan* (NHS England, 2019). A particular focus of the campaign was to recruit people with no previous experience of care. Activities included a national recruitment campaign (called *'We Are The NHS'*), the development of the *Accelerated Care Certificate* programme (discussed below) and a website dedicated to solely to support worker role vacancies, which also pre-screened candidates for employers. The campaign recognised that raising awareness of support worker careers was key to its success (see Chapter 3).

Although there is very little evidence available about how newly recruited support workers feel in the early days of their employment, it is reasonable to suppose that people joining these roles for the first time may experience a 'shock' similar to that experienced by newly qualified nurses On-boarding, though, is not just important for new employees, it is also allows employers to be assured that the people who work for them have the right values, attitudes and capabilities.

The term 'on-boarding' is sometimes, but incorrectly, used synonymously with 'induction'. It is though a much broader term that encompasses:

- Attracting candidates.
- Recruitment and selection.
- Appointment.
- Induction.
- Initial training and appraisal.

The programmes we discussed in the previous chapter, such as volunteering, internships and work experience, can also be seen as part of on-boarding, as they are means of allowing potential recruits to get a 'taste' of healthcare employment and workplaces. They also allow groups who may be disadvantaged in the labour market to gather experience to assist them apply for work and enter employment. Across all the elements of on-boarding there is a need to ensure that an inclusive approach is taken. The on-boarding requirements of a newly employed support worker who has a disability or who has experienced long periods of unemployment for example, will be different to an adult career changer or someone recruited directly from school after finishing their A levels.

Although there is a paucity of evidence about the impact of the early experience of work on decisions by new employees to remain in or quit a role (Buchan et al., 2019), it appears that early experiences, which begins even before the application stage, can be significant (Acevdeo and Yancey, 2011). Camilla Cavendish (2013) in her review reported on an outreach programme run by a NHS trust in Yorkshire which was aimed at potential support worker recruits and comprised open days during which potential applicants had the chance to see the hospital and meet other staff, as well as receive information about working as a support worker. Linked to the open days was an extended induction programme and a buddy system. Cavendish (ibid.) reported that this comprehensive approach resulted in turnover rates for new recruits falling from 17% to 12%, sickness absence from 8% to 5% and delivered a 100% attendance rate at interviews.

We do have some evidence of what the experience of new recruits to NHS support worker roles is like. In 2021, 379 newly appointed support workers recruited by trusts in Yorkshire and the North East (NHS Employers, 2021) were surveyed. This found that:

- A minority (10%) experienced long delays (16 weeks) between being short listed and commencing employment.
- One in ten of the support workers (who were employed in 13 separate trusts) were unaware of *The Care Certificate*.
- Less than half (45%) felt informed about their future career and skill development opportunities open to them.

BOX 4.2 THE IMPACT OF 12-HOUR SHIFTS

An issue often considered to be a factor influencing turnover rates in the NHS, including for support workers, is the impact of 12-hour shifts (see Cavendish, 2013, for example). In a small-scale study (n = 25) based on interviews, Thomson and Hare Duke (2015) explored attitudes towards working long shifts and found mixed results amongst the support workers they talked too. The support workers in the study identified both negative and positive consequences arising from shift working. Negatives were that the staff felt fatigued, which some felt might impact on patient care (for example on their ability to be observant), and also that they had poor work-life balance. However, the study also found that support staff had positive views about undertaking long shifts. They reported that care might be improved due to greater continuity and having more time to complete tasks. Moreover, support workers reported a sense of 'satisfaction in working hard and getting things done' (p. 14).

There are several costs for NHS employers resulting from high turnover (McKee and Ashton, 2004; Jones et al., 2007):

- Advertising and recruitment costs.
- Vacancy costs (such as agency costs, overtime, closed beds, hospital diversions).
- Repeated orientation and training.
- Decreased productivity.
- Loss of organisational knowledge.
- Increased workload for existing staff which may result in absenteeism and may impact on organisational culture and the quality of care.

We will now consider the various elements comprising on-boarding starting with recruitment and selection.

Recruitment and selection

The process of getting on-boarding right begins before vacancies are even advertised. There is much excellent information and guidance on recruitment and selection (NHS Employers, 2022). NHS trusts should have recruitment policies and employ recruitment managers. The aim here is to provide a brief overview of approaches that can be taken but also to offer insights into how recruitment and selection can be incorporated into Outside/In GYO workforce approaches and address some of the issues that may lead to staff quitting in the early days of employment.

Recruitment and selection comprise the following steps:

1. Defining the role.
2. Attracting the candidates.
3. The application and selection process.
4. Appointment.

The Cavendish Review (2013) recommended that senior staff, such as Directors of Nursing, be more involved in the process of recruiting and selecting support workers. Whoever is involved in the process should have the necessary training including on how to avoid bias. Thought should also be given to involving service users in the process.

Defining the role

The quality and consistency of support worker job descriptions and person specifications varies. This can be a consequence of poor job design (see Chapters 1 and 2). By way of illustration when writing this section, I looked on the *NHS Jobs* website and searched for vacancies at band 3 for nursing support workers. Below are the first three results (there were 472 vacancies in total when I looked) and the education requirements they specify as 'essential'.

Job 1

- Evidence of general education e.g. GCSE's or equivalent.
- NVQ III in Health care or equivalent qualification.
- HEE Care Certificate.

Job 2

- Have proficiency in English and Maths and pass the trust Maths and English test on interview.
- Have at least five pass grades GCSEs or equivalent.

Job 3

- Good basic education.
- NVQ level 3 in Health and Social Care or equivalent experience / qualifications.

Remember these are all general nursing support roles and all graded at *Agenda for Change* band 3. Besides the inconsistency of entry-requirements a number of other points could be made. NVQs ended in 2015. Their inclusion is probably a reflection of the fact that they were, in 2022, still listed on many *Job Profiles* for support workers. They were occupationally based so the two posts asking for a NVQ level 3 will exclude external candidates such as healthcare BTEC students.

Some requirements are vague. What does 'proficiency' in English and Maths mean, and actually would not possession of GCSEs indicate proficiency and, if so, why also ask the candidate to pass a test at interview? The question could also be asked, which we address below, to what extent have efforts been made to make job information and selection processes accessible?

Vacancies are, then, an opportunity to review job descriptions, to ensure that they are up-to-date – including qualification requirements, accurate, consistent and include only job relevant tasks, responsibilities and requirements. Where possible, job descriptions and person specifications should be mapped against the appropriate occupational competency frameworks, which are discussed in the next chapter. Part of the review process should comprise a check that the job is appropriately graded for its responsibilities. Furthermore, NHS England's (2020) *Our NHS People Promise* includes a commitment to support flexible working. Organisations need to consider when designing roles how they can support flexible working, such as job shares and part-time working. Consideration should also be given at an early stage to any adjustments that could be made to assist potential recruits who may need additional support. Working with agencies that support those who experience barriers to work will assist this.

Attracting the candidates

In the context of Outside/In GYO workforce strategies the process of attracting candidates includes actively targeting groups that are underrepresented in the workforce. This will involve, in part, using the local labour market interventions discussed in the last chapter (such as engaging with colleges and schools). In recruitment process terms this means making clear in job adverts applications from such candidates are particularly welcome as well as working with specialist employment agencies or charities and voluntary organisations to actively seek and support people into NHS jobs.

In addition to the various interventions associated with Outside/In GYO workforce strategies, local recruitment campaign to attract people into support worker or other roles could be organised. In North West London when we realised that a large number of healthcare BTEC students in local colleges were not entering health or social care employment, recruitment fairs were held, that included general practices, to raise awareness of the opportunities available. Other job marketing activities designed at engaging with local labour markets, include open days and career related events. There are a number of 'celebration' days held, including ones specifically aimed at NHS support workers often organised by professional bodies and trade unions (like the RCM's *MSW Week*); as well as more general work-related ones such as *National Apprenticeship Week*. These can be useful to link a campaign or event too. Working with Job Centre Plus and the National Careers Service will also help them signpost and support candidates to NHS jobs locally.

Consideration needs to be given as to *where* adverts are placed. Just using traditional routes, particularly *the NHS Jobs* website may well mean employers are not maximising their potential talent pool. Take care leavers, as an example. There are over 70,000 care leavers in this country at any one time. Looked after young people are three times more likely to be Not in Employment, Education or Training when they leave the care system. This is largely because they have not had the same life experiences, such as positive role models, as other young people (Learning and Work Institute, 2017). Care leavers are a group the NHS should actively seek to recruit, for the reasons set out in the last chapter. Doing so, though, will require not only making clear in advertisement and job material that applications from care leavers are positively welcomed, but also thinking about where looked after young people and care leavers might see adverts. Local authority teams can assist with this. Given their life experiences, some care leavers may require additional support in understanding job descriptions and what might be expected of them at work (this is where pre-employment programmes, such as job shadowing, and links with specialist employment agencies are valuable). The job brokerage system (below) is a means of comprehensively addressing barriers such as these.

Support worker vacancies are also an opportunity for existing staff to develop their careers either through moving to a higher graded role with more responsibility or moving across into other NHS support occupation. Recall that a common route for support workers employed in primary care is to start working as a receptionist in a practice. Consideration should be given to whether a vacancy can be filled internally or offered as a secondment. This should though be done in the context of an assessment of the diversity of the workforce that includes an understanding of who is being promoted. One trust, for example, found that although the majority of its staff were from BAME backgrounds, the majority of promoted staff were not (NHS Employers, 2020).

Application and selection

Whatever application process (such as CV, application forms and assessment centres) is used, it needs to be ensured that it does not discriminate. This means ensuring that people with disabilities, such as those who are visually impaired or may benefit from an Easy Reader application, can access job information and the application process and that open recruitment processes are adopted that do not create barriers for disadvantaged groups. All applicants need to be assessed fairly so that no one is discriminated against due to their gender, age, disability, religion or sexual orientation, for example. This can include taking positive action such as guaranteeing interviews to any applicant who meets the *minimum* job requirement or who is disabled or a care leaver or using a job brokerage system to support people into NHS work, for example.

Appointment

It is important that interviews are also carried out in an inclusive way. This will mean making some adjustments for certain groups. Taking care leavers as an example again, the Learning and Work Institute (2017) provide useful advice on how interviews can be conducted in a supportive way:

- Interviews should be conducted in an informal and semi-structured way.
- A variety of interview techniques should be used to judge whether to appoint or not, such as questions and answers, role play, tasks and exercises. This will allow people to show case their strengths.
- Care leavers (and other disadvantaged groups) do not compete for jobs on an even playing find and so may require additional support throughout the recruitment process, such as:
  - Letting candidates know what might be expected of them at interviews.
  - Carrying out mock interviews.
  - Letting candidates know what is expected of them in terms of appearance and presentation.
  - Calling them the day of the interview to provide encouragement.
- Interviewers should not have pre-conceptions. A candidate whose appearance may not be to the standard expected may not be projecting her attitude to the job or work, but rather reflecting her personal circumstances.

Good practice means that feedback is given to all candidates who are interviewed, but also feedback is sought *from* candidates about their experience of applying. This will, amongst other things, provide employers with insights into their processes but also how their organisation is perceived (as an employer) by the local community.

The delay between an interview, an offer of appointment and starting work should be as short as possible and the induction process start as soon as possible once an offer of employment is made.

BOX 4.3 VALUE BASED RECRUITMENT (VBR)

In 2014 HEE published a framework to assist organisations assess whether the values of candidates applying for jobs, aligned with the values of the *NHS Constitution* (which are: (1) working together for patients, (2) respect and diversity, (3) commitment to quality of care, (4) compassion, (5) improving lives and (6) everyone counts). Values matter because they drive behaviours and actions. The HEE framework included six core requirements:

1. Employer values should be mapped against the *NHS Constitution*.
2. Service users should be involved in the recruitment process, at some point.
3. NHS values should be prominent in job material including marketing.
4. Candidate's values should be assessed in interviews.
5. All candidates should receive feedback following their interview.
6. NHS values should be embedded in new employee's induction. The framework includes a reference to *The Care Certificate* one aim of which is to ensure support staff have the right values to work in healthcare.

There may be a number of reasons why some people are not shortlisted for support worker roles or fail at interview. For example, they may not have attained sufficient functional skills. Recall the job advert above that required candidates to pass a functional skills test at interview. An increasing number of trusts are 'holding' such candidates and identifying ways that they can be assisted to successfully gain employment in the future. One of the advantages of the job brokerage approach adopted in North West London is that, working with local colleges and others, candidates are supported prior to application and appointment.

A new model of NHS recruitment for support workers – job brokerage

Job brokerage is an approach to recruitment and employment that brings together specialist employment agencies, and others such as council Health and Work programme leads, with employers and potential candidates. Candidates are matched with vacancies, supported in their application (for example with CV writing or employability skills training) and screened so employers see 'role ready' candidates (Murphy, 2019).

The North West London ICS utilised the model with West London local authorities to recruit the workforce for the Covid-19 mass vaccination centres in 2020, but more widely because of its aspiration to address workforce shortages through recruiting more local people, including those most distant from employment. Describing the approach David Francis, Director of the WLA told me that a

> large consortium of employment, skills and health partners came together with one goal: to achieve positive outcomes for local residents by supporting the NHS Mass Vaccination Programme, whilst making best use of public money and integrating public, private and voluntary organisations. Partners largely refocused existing employment support budgets to ensure that the required resources were deployed to make this project a success ... Where local authorities did not have existing services to support this project, WLA's wide network of voluntary and charity organisation and private health and employment providers seconded resource into the project to support.

The rapid recruitment of the workforce needed to staff the nine West London mass vaccination centres was organised by the local authorities along with other partners, including the voluntary sector and employment agencies. Recruitment created opportunities for local people who were either unemployed or furloughed to gain employment or work experience. Nearly 4,500 local people applied for roles, 60% from BAME communities, with 1,911 being finally deployed.

Towards the end of 2020 the NHS needed to recruit people quickly to mass vaccination centre roles to help vaccinate over 2 million people in West

London. The need for speed enabled the development of a simple recruitment process that could reach into local communities and find suitable people to fill the administrative and vaccinator roles in centres.

Kim Archer, Head of the WLA Work and Health Programme, told me.

It was decided early on that the ICS would seek to retain as many of vaccination workforce as possible once the centres closed. An unpublished survey conducted by the ICS in the summer of 2021 found that 40% of the workforce wished to continue to work in healthcare – over half of these in a clinical role. In response, the ICS and West London local authorities established a process to these staff into NHS trust vacancies. The process had four steps:

1. Engagement with the vaccination workforce via road shows, survey, and a weekly newsletter.
2. Career advisors assist staff as the centres closed.
3. A central recruitment team that matched potential candidates (taking account of their skills, location, and areas of interest) with local vacancies. This screening process was previously undertaken by NHS trust recruitment teams.
4. Candidates applied for vacancies with suitable candidates interviewed. This process was streamlined compared to the normal NHS application process. If no candidates were suitable for the role, vacancies moved to open advertising

It was estimated by the WLA that the process saved the NHS an equivalent if £2 million in recruitment costs.

Planned prior to Covid-19, and organised in a similar way to the vaccination job brokerage recruitment process described above, the ICS, West London local authorities and partners designed a small pilot job brokerage programme with three NHS trusts – Imperial College Healthcare NHS Trust, London North West University Healthcare NHS Trust and West London NHS Trust. This approach targeted local long term unemployed people, helping them to transition, with support, into NHS employment. The normal NHS recruitment and application process was streamlined and external partners, including The Shaw Trust, were used to identify and support unemployed residents. First run in early 2021 the pilot resulted in the employment of 19 people – more than originally intended (due to the quality of candidates). Imperial College Healthcare NHS Trust subsequently adopted the approach as its primary source for entry-level recruitment. The job brokerage was linked to an employment skills education programme, that also included elements of *The Care Certificate,* co-developed with NHS employers, delivered by local colleges, and funded by the devolved London Adult Education Budget.

A job brokerage model has a number of advantages for the NHS. It can find and support under-represented groups into NHS jobs. It can help the NHS workforce to reflect its local communities. It can create partnerships with a number of local labour market organisations and it can reduce recruitment costs.

Induction

Induction is the process by which new starters initially become familiar with an organisation, its ways of working and culture (Noon and Heery, 2017). The CIPD (2021) highlight the benefits arising from an effective induction process as:

- The new employee settles in quickly.
- The new employee integrates into their team.
- The new employee understands the organisation's values and culture.
- As a result of the above, new employees become productive faster.
- Turnover is reduced.

Induction begins even before a new support worker steps foot into a hospital, surgery, clinic or community setting. Pre-employment communications are a vital first step in the induction process and might include providing the new employee with joining instructions, site plans, transport information, a welcome pack and other relevant documentation. A newly recruited support worker who has not worked in a care setting before may be feeling anxious about their future role and hospitals, in particular, can be daunting places to work in if you are not familiar with them. This pre-employment induction stage can help alleviate some of that anxiety.

What makes induction successful for a support worker is no different to what makes it successful for a new doctor, nurse or radiographer (CIPD, 2021, and NHS Employers, 2021). Induction should:

- Take account of whether the new support worker has previous experience of NHS employment or not.
- Provide information in a measured way. It is important not to overload new starters with too much information, too quickly.
- Ensure a range of people contribute to induction including HR, peers, managers – and the chief executive.
- Provide new starters with an up-to-date job description.
- Provide details of the appraisal and development process, along with future opportunities to develop, including study leave policies and funding.
- Tell new starters how to access information, including through digital platforms.
- Provide information and guidance on pay, terms and conditions, health and safety, patient safety, equality, diversity and inclusion, annual leave, sick leave and freedom of information policies.
- Provide information on operating practices including rotas, shift handover arrangements and supervision.
- Include a tour of the department and facilitate the meeting of staff. A 'buddy' should be provided to help orientation and socialisation. Peer-to-peer support should be considered.

- New staff should be told clearly about the organisation's values and the expectations of them. For support workers this will include the *Code of Practice* (see Box 4.4 below) and will be reinforced through completion of *The Care Certificate* shortly after commencing employment.

BOX 4.4 CODE OF CONDUCT FOR HEALTHCARE AND ADULT SOCIAL CARE SUPPORT WORKERS

In response to the Cavendish Review (2013), Skills for Health published a *Code of Conduct for Healthcare and Adult Social Care Support Workers* which comprised the following standards for support staff:

1. Should be accountable by making sure they are able to answer for their actions or omissions.
2. Must promote and uphold the privacy, dignity, rights, health and wellbeing of people who use health and care services and their carers at all times.
3. Work in collaboration with colleagues to ensure the delivery of high-quality, safe and compassionate healthcare, and support.
4. Communicate in an open and effective way to promote the health, safety and wellbeing of people who use health and care services and their carers.
5. Respect a person's right to confidentiality.
6. Strive to improve the quality of healthcare, care and support through continuing professional development.
7. Uphold and promote equality, diversity and inclusion.

The Care Certificate

Following initial statutory and mandatory training, the first developmental opportunity NHS clinical support staff should access is *The Care Certificate*, either as a stand-alone induction programme or as part of an apprenticeship. *The Care Certificate* is a national set of 15 standards that were introduced following the recommendations of the Cavendish Review (2013) and developed by HEE, Skills for Health and Skills for Care. It should be completed by all patient-facing support workers in the NHS.

Cavendish (ibid.) set out two objectives for *The Care Certificate* (which she originally called the *Certificate of Fundamental Care*). Firstly, she wished to ensure that all service facing support workers in health and social care had the necessary fundamental knowledge, skills, and behaviours to deliver quality care. Secondly, and in response to her review's finding that support worker learning and development was not consistent, she wished to support transferable learning across the workforce. It was further hoped, by others, that *The Care Certificate* would also support effective and safe delegation of tasks by registered staff (Glasper, 2013) and, through the application of common national standards, contribute to the regulation of support workers (Hayes et al., 2015).

BOX 4.5 *THE CARE CERTIFICATE* – **THE DETAILS**

The Care Certificate comprises 15 standards (see below) which all new service-user facing support workers should complete on employment. *The Care Certificate* cannot be partly completed. Existing staff are also able to complete *The Care Certificate,* although the extent to which they have done so varies by employer (Thomas et al., 2018). The apprenticeship standards relevant to clinical support staff all include *The Care Certificate* within them, although if an apprentice has previously completed *The Care Certificate,* they are not required to re-study it.

The Care Certificate standards are:

1. Understand your role.
2. Your personal development.
3. Duty of care.
4. Equality and diversity.
5. Work in a person-centred way.
6. Communication.
7. Privacy and dignity.
8. Fluids and nutrition.
9. Awareness of mental health, dementia and learning disabilities.
10. Safeguarding adults.
11. Safeguarding children.
12. Basic life support.
13. Health and safety.
14. Handling information.
15. Infection prevention and control.

Each standard includes a series of individual outcomes and, for each of these, details of what staff are expected to have learnt to aid assessment. For example, the *Communication* standard's first outcome is – *Understanding the importance of effective communication at work.* To be successfully assessed against this standard staff need to demonstrate that they can describe the different ways that people communicate, how communications affect relations at work and why it is important to observe people's reactions when communicating to them.

Staff must complete all 15 standards through a combination of learning and practice. Learning may take place through instruction, self-directed learning and/or with work-based mentors, through the application of learning in practice. Staff are assessed as to whether they have met the standards by an 'occupationally competent person'. Until support workers have completed *The Care Certificate* new staff must work under close supervision. Whilst mapped against National Occupational Standards, *The Care Certificate* is not a formal qualification.

Unusually for support workforce initiatives, there is a body of research investigating *The Care Certificate* (Bradley, 2017). Although not mandatory, (despite both Cavendish's (2013) and Willis's (2015) recommendation that it should be), the introduction of *The Care Certificate* in the NHS has been extensive amongst NHS trusts (see Box 4.6 for a discussion of its implementation in primary care). Thomas and colleagues (2018) found that 97% of NHS trusts had in fact implemented it. However, whilst *The Care Certificate* exists in almost all NHS trusts, individual employee access to it may be uneven. Kessler and colleagues (2021 and 2022) survey of nursing support staff found that 26% of the sample had *not* undertaken *The Care Certificate* – although almost all *new* recruits had, as part of their induction. Griffin (2021) found that almost half of support workers employed in mental health services had not completed *The Care Certificate* with a quarter being unaware that it existed, whilst in maternity services 43% had not completed it (Griffin, 2018).

'Implementation' of *The Care Certificate*, Thomas and colleagues (2018) wrote, had resulted in a 'generally positive impact on…organisations, staff and those in receipt of care' (p. 85). Thomas and colleagues (ibid.) and Haigh and Garside (2019) both found evidence that completion increased staff confidence. Gilding (2017) found that both support staff and clinical educators valued *The Care Certificate* as a development tool. Gilding's (ibid.) study, although small scale, found that *The Care Certificate* assisted support staff to reflect on their role, improved team working and helped clarify role boundaries, as well as increasing occupational knowledge.

Thomas and colleagues (2018) found that organisations felt the content of *The Care Certificate* was relevant to practice, Rodgers and colleagues (2019), though, suggest that whilst its standards address ethical issues such as safeguarding, as a whole it 'does not teach ethical theory or moral distress' (p. 2311). Moral distress is the 'psychological distress that can develop in response to a morally challenging event' (ibid., 2306). This, they argued, is a particular issue for NHS support staff because they can frequently feel powerless in such situations compared to registered staff. Given the issue of 'transition shock' touched on above that support staff may face when entering healthcare roles for the first time, we may conjecture that this could be a significant omission – not just form *The Care Certificate* but support worker learning and development more widely.

BOX 4.6 *THE CARE CERTIFICATE* AND GENERAL PRACTICE

The Care Certificate applies to all health and social care settings including support workers employed in general practice. Both the Care Quality Commission (the independent NHS regulator) and British Medical Association recommend practices implement it. In primary care settings assessors are likely to be Practice Managers or Practice Nurses, although they could, as in other areas, be another experienced support worker. General practices have faced two challenges implementing *The Care Certificate*. Firstly, the need for it to be contextualised to primary care and secondly, capacity to provide learning and assessment. On the first point guidance has been produced (Health Education Thames Valley and Institute of Vocational Leaning and Workforce Research, n.d., for example). On the second there are a number of options to increase capacity. Practices within PCNs can combine to share learning and assessment, use can be made of online learning resources or links could be made to local NHS trusts to access their training resources, although again it will be important to ensure that learning is relevant to primary care. Support worker apprenticeships at RQF levels 2 and 3 include *The Care Certificate* so there is an opportunity for practices to recruit people as apprentices so that they achieve it, through that route, rather than a standalone programme.

The main issues research has identified associated with the implementation of *The Care Certificate* relate to the second objective Cavendish (2013) had for it –transferability. These issues were summarised by Argyle and colleagues (2020) as: 'the extent of variation in the implementation of the Care Certificate, potential barriers to implementation, how delivery methods differ and how possession of the Care Certificate, which should be transferable between employers, affects staff mobility' (pp. 514–515). Gilding's (2017) study found variations in the assistance that staff completing the Certificate received within a *single* NHS trust. The reasons for this variability were – availability of time off to study, support from teams and whether supervisors were familiar with the areas *The Care Certificate* covered. Thomas and colleagues (2018) identified lack of capacity and a lack of sanctions for non-implementation as the main barriers to implementation. Gilding (2017) recommended that there should be national guidance on support, given its importance in assisting staff to complete *The Care Certificate* and orientate as part of their induction. Ashurst (2016) also stressed the importance of support for new starters completing *The Care Certificate*.

In their evaluation of the early introduction of the *The Care Certificate* in health and social care, Thomas and colleagues (2018) identified a series of features which characterised successful implementation. The features below might easily be applied to support worker education and training more generally:

1. Leaders recognise of the importance of training and development.
2. There are members of staff dedicated to overseeing staff training and development.
3. Integration of *The Care Certificate* into existing training and induction programmes.
4. A blended, holistic, practical, and participatory approach to delivery of the training.
5. Application of *The Care Certificate* to existing staff as well as new recruits.
6. Peer and mentoring support for staff completing *The Care Certificate*.
7. Adjustment of materials and assessments for staff facing literacy or language barriers.
8. Regular communications.

BOX 4.7 *THE ACCELERATED CARE CERTIFICATE (ACC)*

Originally staff were expected to complete *The Care Certificate* within three months of starting work, although actual completion times vary considerably between employers (Thomas et al., 2018). The impact of Covid-19, including reduced opportunities to carry out face-to-face teaching, led to employers placing a greater emphasis on on-line learning (Connor, 2020), and in 2021 the creation of the ACC as part of NHS England's *HCSW2020* campaign. The ACC seeks to shorten the period of time between when people apply to work in the NHS and, if successful, are judged to be occupationally competent through completion of *The Care Certificate*. It is in effect, an accelerated recruitment and induction process. In summary the ACC involves candidates self-assessing against the Care Certificate prior to employment and then being assessed at interviews through the asking of Certificate-related questions. On appointment candidates are assigned a mentor and sent an induction pack, whilst their references are obtained, DBS checks organised and occupational health assessments organised. Candidates may commence the theory-based elements of *The Care Certificate* via *eLearning for Health*'s on-line modules. Once in employment they continue learning through a blended approach including with their mentor. They are assessed through online and work-based methods. They will also complete induction statutory and mandatory training. The ACC takes between four and six weeks to complete

---

It appears that concerns initially expressed that *The Care Certificate* would become a 'tick box' exercise (Peate, 2015) were unfounded. However, leaving the details of implementation to individual employers has impacted on transferability (Peate, 2015; Gilding, 2017). Thomas and colleagues (2018) 'found the Care Certificate was rarely used as a fully portable, standardised training certificate' due to employer 'scepticism about the quality of prior training' (pp. 85 and 86). This has also meant that a *potential* consequence of *The Care Certificate* – as a means to regulate support staff through national common standards (Hayes et al., 2015) – has not materialised.

Conclusion

Successful on-boarding delivers a number of benefits ranging from attracting the right candidates to roles, inducting newly recruited staff into an organisation and its ways of working, and providing new staff with the necessary knowledge, skills and behaviours to do their job safely and effectively. Although taking place over a relatively short period of time – although longer than is sometimes thought – on-boarding is an important process than determines whether a new employer remains with an organisation or not. What evidence there is, suggests that the NHS does not always get this right for newly employed support workers including insufficiently recognising the apprehension they may feel moving into a patient care role for the first time and failing to communicate to new recruits about how they can progress their careers in the future. *The Care Certificate* has an important and positive role to play in on-boarding new support staff.

On-boarding is a key component of Outside/In GYP workforce strategies – helping to bring people from outside NHS organisations into them, including those who may be underrepresented in the workforce. The rest of this book is concerned with what happens once support staff are employed and how their contribution to care can be maximised and how they care develop their careers.

Checklist

- On-boarding is a process that starts with prior to recruitment and continues through the first year of employment. Each step needs to be linked, inclusive and appropriately supported – is this the case?
- Is there high turnover amongst support worker roles? If so, are the reasons for this understood? How can turnover be reduced?
- Are 'stay' interviews undertaken with new recruits after their first year of employment to gain their insights into the on-boarding process and organisation more generally?
- Is anything known about how the local community perceives the NHS as an employer?
- Consider a job brokerage approach to recruit into support roles. This will involve working with local labour market partners as discussed in the last chapter.
- Review interview candidate selection and interview processes in light of potential recruits who might be disadvantaged.
- Limit, as far as possible, the time between a job offer and starting work.
- Provide pastural support for new starters such as mentors/buddies.
- Ensure *The Care Certificate*'s delivery is sufficiently supported and that it is integrated into the induction process and training more generally.
- Recognise that new starters without experience of healthcare may be anxious and might require support due to the physical and mental demands of the roles.
- Support workers should be able from day one of employment understand the opportunities that are available for them to develop their careers over time, including how they will access learning.

References

Acevedo, J. M. and Yancey, G. B. (2011). Assessing new employee orientation programs. *Journal of Workplace Learning* 23(5), 349–354.

Argyle, E., Thomson, T., Arthur, A., Maben, J., Schneider, J. and Wharrad, H. (2020). Introducing the Care Certificate Evaluation: Innovative practice. *Dementia* 19(2), 512–517.

Ashurst, A. (2016). Implementing the Care Certificate: Supporting new staff. *Nursing and Residential Care* 18(10), 568–569.

Bradley, P. (2017). Have a care. *British Journal of Healthcare Assistants* 11(5), 213.

Buchan, J., Charlesworth, A., Gershlick, B. and Seccombe, I. (2019). *A Critical Moment: NHS Staffing Trends, Retention and Attrition.* Health Foundation. Available from: www.health.org. uk/sites/default/files/upload/publications/2019/A%20Critical%20Moment_1.pdf

Cavendish, C. (2013). *Cavendish Review. An Independent Enquiry into Healthcare Assistants and Support Workers in the NHS and Social Care Settings.* London, Department of Health. Available from: https://assets.publishing.service.gov.uk/government/uploads/system/uploads/attachment_data/file/236212/Cavendish_Review.pdf

Cavendish, C. (2021). The NHS faces a bleak midwinter as its staffing crisis hits home. *The Financial Times*, 17 December 2021. Available from: www.ft.com/content/8f177676-4496-4aff-a726-74ef3210c905

CIPD (2020). Induction. Fact Sheet. Available from: www.cipd.co.uk/knowledge/funda mentals/people/recruitment/induction-factsheet#gref

Connor, J. (2020). The Care Certificate…but condensed. *British Journal of Healthcare Assistants* 14(8), 398–399.

Finlayson, B., Dixon, J., Meadows, S. and Blair, G. (2002) 'Mind the gap': the extent of the NHS nursing shortage. *BMJ*, 7 September 2002; 325(7363): 538–541.

Gilding, M. (2017). Implementing the Care Certificate: A development tool or a tick box exercise? *British Journal of Healthcare Assistants* 11(5), 242–248.

Glasper, A. (2010). Widening participation in pre-registration nursing. *British Journal of Nursing* 19(4), 924–925.

Griffin, R. (2018). *The Deployment, Education and Development of Maternity Support Workers in England. A Scoping Report to Health Education England.* RCM, available from: www.rcm. org.uk/media/2347/the-deployment-education-and-development-of-maternity-supp ort-workers-in-england.pdf

Griffin, R. (2021). *A Rewarding Job, but Frustrating Career. The Education, Development, and Deployment of Clinical Support Workers Employed in NHS Mental Health Services.* London: King's College London.

Haigh, S. M. and Garside, J. (2019) Effects of the Care Certificate on healthcare assistants' ability to identify and manage deteriorating patients. *British Journal of Healthcare Assistants* 26(3): 16–20.

Hayes, C., Garfield, I. and Beardmore, P. (2015). Housing a modernisation agenda: ensuring authentic learning environments for healthcare assistants. *British Journal of Healthcare Assistants* 9(2), 84–92.

Health Education Thames Valley and Institute of Vocational Leaning and Workforce Research (n.d.). *Hints and Tips for Assessing the Care Certificate in General Practice.* Health Education Thames Valley. Available from: www.oxfordhealth.nhs.uk/library/wp-content/uploads/sites/3/Hints-and-Tips-for-GPs-assessing-the-Care-Certificate.pdf

HEE (n.d.). *Growing the Numbers. Literature Review on Nurses Leaving the NHS.* Available from: www.hee.nhs.uk/sites/default/files/documents/Nurses%20leaving%20pract ice%20-%20Literature%20Review.pdf

HEE (2016). *Values Based Recruitment Framework.* Available from: www.hee.nhs.uk/sites/defa ult/files/documents/VBR_Framework%20March%202016.pdf

Jones, B. C. and Gates, M. (2007). The costs and benefits of nurse turnover: A business case for nurse retention. *The Online Journal of Issues in Nursing* 12(3). https://ojin.nursingworld. org/MainMenuCategories/ANAMarketplace/ANAPeriodicals/OJIN/TableofConte nts/Volume122007/No3Sept07/NurseRetention.html

Kessler, I., Steils, N., Esser, A. and Grant, D. (2021) Understanding career development and progression from a healthcare support worker perspective Part 1. *British Journal of Healthcare Assistants* 15(11), 526–531. https://doi.org/10.12968/bjha.2021.15.11.526

Kessler, I., Steils, N., Esser, A. and Grant, D. (2022). Understanding career development and progression from a healthcare support worker perspective Part 2. *British Journal of Healthcare Assistants* 16(1), 6–10. https://doi.org/10.12968/bjha.2022.16.1.6

Learning and Work Institute (2017). *Building Successful Careers: Employer Guide to Supporting Care Leavers in the Workplace.* https://learningandwork.org.uk/wp-content/uploads/2020/05/Building-successful-careers-Employer-guide-to-supporting-care-leavers-in-the-workplace.pdf

McKee, M. G. and Ashton, K. (2004). Stresses of daily life, in: Lang, R. and Hensrud, D. D. (eds), *Clinical Preventive Medicine*, 3rd ed. Chicago, IL: AMA Press, pp. 81–91.

Murphy, H. (2019). *Job Brokerage in In-Work Progression Programmes. Learning and Work Foundation.* Available from: www.walcotfoundation.org.uk/uploads/1/7/2/2/17226772/job-brokerage-in-inwork-progression.pdf

NHS Employers (2020). *Promotion, Praise and Promise: West London NHS Trust.* Available from: www.nhsemployers.org/case-studies/promotion-praise-and-promise

NHS Employers (2021). *SAS Induction Checklist.* Available from: www.nhsemployers.org/articles/sas-induction-checklist

NHS Employers (2021). Optimising attraction, recruitment, support and career development for new Healthcare Support Workers. NHS employers surveyed newly appointed healthcare support workers (HCSWs) in the North East and Yorkshire Region. Available from: www.nhsemployers.org/articles/optimising-attraction-recruitment-support-and-career-development-new-healthcare-support

NHS Employers (2022). Recruitment and workforce supply. Supporting you to attract and recruit staff from the UK and abroad, to develop a sustainable workforce. Available from: www.nhsemployers.org/recruitment

NHS England (2019). *The NHS Long Term Plan.* Available from: www.longtermplan.nhs.uk

NHS England (2020). *Our NHS People Promise.* Available from: www.england.nhs.uk/ournhspeople/online-version/lfaop/our-nhs-people-promise/

Noon, M. and Heery, M. (2017). *A Dictionary of Human Resource Management.* Oxford. Oxford University Press.

Peate, I. (2015). The Care Certificate: Not worth the paper it is written on? *British Journal of Healthcare Assistants* 9(12), 583–584.

Rodger, D., Blackshaw, B. and Young, A. (2015). Moral distress in healthcare assistants: A discussion with recommendations. *Nursing Ethics* 26(8–8), 2306–2313.

Thomas, L. and Hare Duke, L. (2015). *The Impact of 12 Hour Shifts on Health Care Assistants: Exploratory Interviews Study.* Institute of Mental Health. Nottingham University. www.england.nhs.uk/6cs/wp-content/uploads/sites/25/2015/09/hca-12h-shifts-interview-study.pdf

Thomas, L., Argyle, E., Khan, Z., Scheider, J., Arthur, A., Mabett, J., Wharrad, H., Guo, B. and Eve, J. (2018). *Evaluating the Care Certificate: A Cross Sector Solution to Assuring Fundamental Skills in Caring.* Department of Health. Policy Research Project.

Wakefield, E. (2018). Is your graduate nurse suffering from transition shock?, *Journal of Perioperative Nursing*, 31(1). https://doi.org/10.26550/2209-1092.1024

Willis, P. (2015). *Raising the Bar: Shape of Caring, A Review of the Future Education and Training of Registered Nurses and Care Assistants.* Available from: www.hee.nhs.uk/sites/default/files/documents/2348-Shape-of-caring-review-FINAL.pdf

PART III
Get on

5

THE BEST YOU CAN BE

Unleashing potential through in-work development and good people management

Introduction

Workforce planning has two elements. The first is ensuring that an organisation has the right numbers of employees. The second is ensuring that the capabilities of those employees are maximised. Kessler (2017) points out that 'it is certainly the case that the management of employees in the healthcare sector has consequences of a distinctive order related to the quality and longevity of life and, more specifically, to the well-being of its most needy and vulnerable citizens: the acute and chronically ill' (p. 311). The *Talent for Care* (HEE, 2014) support workforce strategy described the objective of its Get On section as making 'sure that people are confident and supported to be *the best that they can be* in their job' (p. 16, emphasis added).

In this chapter we move on to the Get On stage of the career cycle, or in GYO terms the In-work Development stage. Get On is about how staff can be enabled to work to their full potential *within their current role*. We will consider the evidence for the impact of human resource interventions, such as appraisals, on staff and service outcomes. There is a growing body of evidence, including from the NHS, showing that employees who experience good people management are more satisfied and deliver positive organisational outcomes (Boorman, 2009; Ogbonnaya and Daniels, 2017; West and Dawson, 2012; Bellet et al., 2019; Evans et al., 2020). Good people management allows staff to 'be the best they can' and to 'thrive' (Evans et al., 2020). This, though, requires addressing *all* the factors that constitute 'good work' including job design, supportive management and access to education and career development opportunities (Ogbonnaya and Daniels, 2017). 'Employees are looking for jobs with better, stronger career trajectories. They desire both recognition and development. Smart companies find ways to reward people by promoting them not only into new roles but also into additional levels within their existing ones' (Mckinsey, 2021: 10).

DOI: 10.4324/9781003251620-11

Drawing on the results of both the *Workforce Race Equality Standard* (NHS England, 2021a, 2020b) and the NHS's *Workforce Disability Equality Standard* (NHS England, 2021c) along with other research, the importance of creating an inclusive workplace environment for employees and the organisational outcomes: this enables, are reviewed.

Good quality appraisals and development reviews should be at the heart of people management and the NHS appraisal system will be considered, and good practice highlighted. Before formal learning opportunities for support workers are described, the factors that enable learning for support staff and employees more generally are discussed. Finally, returning to Fuller and Unwin's (2011) model of expansive and restrictive learning cultures, the importance of organisational learning is stressed.

The In-work Development stage of GYO workforce strategies is closely linked to the Inside-Up stage, most obviously through appraisals, which allow support staff to identify future development and progression opportunities – a process the NHS does not always get right for its support workers. Given the specific and long-standing issues associated with work-based routes into healthcare degrees – an important element of Inside/Up – this will be considered in Chapter 7.

BOX 5.1 HUMAN RESOURCE MANAGEMENT

The terms 'human resources' (HR) and 'human resource management' (HRM) first emerged in the 1980s (Armstrong, 2012). Many, many words have been written and, journal and book pages filled, with discussions about what HR is, how it differs from management and its impact (see Bratton and Gold, 2019 for example). When discussing HR and HRM, I am referring to a strategic approach to the management, capability, capacity, wellbeing, effort and commitment of an organisation's employees so as to meet organisational goals. HR comprises a range of policies, practices and procedures integrated with other organisational strategies. An example of this, in the context of the NHS was discussed in the last chapter, when the positive impact of providing employment in the NHS (a HR objective) on health inequalities (an NHS service objective) was considered. HR embraces a range of activities, including workforce composition and diversity, retention, skills attainment and pay. HR stresses the importance of people to an organisation's outcomes, success and future survival. Management is part of HR but not the whole story (Armstrong, 2012).

Human Resources and organisational performance in the NHS

This section will review the evidence for the effectiveness of HR in the NHS and the efficacy of individual interventions. There is not space for a wider critique of

NHS HR policy (see Kessler, 2017 for a discussion), but it is worth noting that the publication of the *NHS Interim People Plan* (NHS England, 2019a) was the first explicit national HR strategy for the NHS for over a decade, a telling omission for the UK's largest employer.

HR activities, such as job design, team working, appraisals and line manager support, as well as wider organisational culture, matter. Collectively they shape employee commitment, health and well-being, effort, and consequently organisational performance, including patient outcomes (Kessler, 2017). As *The Boorman Review* (2009) noted the health and well-being of NHS staff is linked to them having 'productive and rewarding jobs' (p. 28). This is not just important for staff but also patients – 'improving the health and well-being of staff is key to enabling the NHS to genuinely provide health and well-being for all' (ibid., 28).

In their seminal study, West and colleagues (2011) analysed data from the 2009 *NHS Staff Survey* to assess whether there was a link between bundles of HR activities designed to increase employee engagement (such as training) and service outcomes. The study found that the 'quality of patient experience...is strongly linked with engagement. Patient satisfaction is significantly higher in trusts with higher level of employee engagement' (West and Dawson, 2012: 19). Other positive outcomes identified were: lower absenteeism and turnover, lower mortality rates and improved patient safety. Reviewing the wider literature West and colleagues (2011) reported, for the NHS, that a 'series of studies...have found relationships between the experience of staff and the experience of patients' (p. 4). *The Boorman Review* (2009) found a link between staff well-being and the following outcomes: absenteeism, turnover, patient satisfaction and infection rates.

Based on self-reported feedback from NHS trusts a review of the NHS appraisal system conducted by the Institute of Employment Studies concluded that appraisals and Personal Development Plans (PDPs) 'contribute directly to patient outcomes' with one NHS trust, for example, finding a clear link between the number of complaints it received and the levels of knowledge and skills staff had as identified through appraisals/PDPs (NHS Staff Council, 2010: 4).

Also reviewing data from the *NHS Staff Survey*, Ogbonnaya and Daniels (2017) found positive links between NHS trusts with extensive HR practices and organisational outcomes. NHS trusts with good people management were:

- More than twice as likely to have staff with high levels of job satisfaction.
- Over three times more likely to have staff with the highest level of engagement, compared to trusts with less extensive talent management practices.
- Over three time more likely to have the lowest level of sickness absence.

Although NHS trusts with good people management practices were over four times as likely to have the most satisfied patients than those that did not, unlike West and colleagues, (2011), Ogbonnaya and Daniels (2017) found no robust statistical evidence for a link between people management practices and patient mortality. Reviewing the wider (non-NHS) literature, Ogbonnaya and Daniels (ibid.) did report that 'high quality work is characterised by job security and well-designed jobs characterised by factors' (p. 6) such as:

- Having input into decisions that affect how, when and what work is accomplished.
- Reasonable work demands and working hours.
- Clear role descriptions.
- Use of skills.
- Variety in tasks.
- Support from co-workers.

To what extent, then, do NHS support workers daily experience of work reflect these features of good work? Unfortunately, in a rare example of the NHS treating its workforce as one, the results of the *NHS Staff Survey* (NHS England and NHS Improvement, 2022) are not broken down by registered and unregistered staff, meaning that it is not possible to compare the experience of support staff with their registered colleagues. The results for the NHS, as a whole, suggest that the workforce is a satisfied one, with only 6% saying that they planned to leave the NHS. This is an improvement from 2018 when 7.5% said they would quit. Whilst staff remain committed to working in healthcare, sizeable numbers are considering leaving their current NHS employer. In 2020, 26% of staff said they 'often' thought about leaving their organisation, one in four that they would 'probably' leave in the next 12 months and 14% that they would leave as soon as they could. This suggests that whilst commitment to the NHS is high amongst health care workers, their commitment to individual employers is less firm. Other results from the national survey suggest the NHS could do more to value their staff, with only just over half (57%) saying they were happy with their opportunities to work flexibly, and just a third saying they thought their employer took positive action in respect of their health and wellbeing. It should be said that staff from BAME communities and those with disabilities (and others) have a less positive experience of work than their white and non-disabled colleagues (Hemmings et al., 2021).

Our review in Chapters 1 and 2 of the experience of support workers in the NHS suggests that they do not always have a positive workplace experience. Recall that many do not feel valued (Griffin, 2021), or are graded fairly (Griffin, 2018), or have access to development opportunities (Cavendish, 2013) or feel they have a 'voice' in their workplace. Clark (2014), for example, reports that nursing support workers are often excluded 'from management discussion leaving them virtually ignored as a group of workers', a consequence of which is that 'local knowledge held by HCAs on patients was not utilised' (p. 309). The unsupportive organisational cultures, Clark (ibid.) found meant that support staff were not able to share knowledge that may have a bearing on patient outcomes. The Nuffield Trust (2021) stressed that the 'role of front line manager is critical to ensuring that clinical support workers are appropriately valued, supervised and held to account' (p. 7).

BOX 5.2 PROCESS THEORY

Process theory suggests that individuals react to their environments. In the context of the workplace many factors might be said to influence NHS staff. These include pay, working conditions, management, the extent to which staff are respected, the extent to which they have access to the learning they need as well as their relationships with colleagues. All these factors impact, for good or bad, on how an individual feels about their job, workplace – and themselves. This in turn has consequences for discretionary effort and commitment, which feeds into to wider organisational outputs some of which are financial (such as turnover rates) and some of which affect patient care. A model of the link between work factors and organisational outputs is shown in Figure 5.1. This could also constitute a Theory of Change for the benefits of investing in support staff.

The Health Foundation (2021) found that lower paid NHS staff had poorer health and wellbeing outcomes than their better paid colleagues due to their working conditions, such as poor access to career progression opportunities. They also did not always feel valued. The Health Foundation (ibid.) made the point that addressing these issues would result not only in positive outcomes for staff but also for the NHS as a whole. The rest of this chapter will consider how to improve people management of support workers, starting with appraisals.

Appraisals

The NHS Constitution for England (Department of Health and Social Care, 2021) pledges states that all NHS staff should have access to personal development,

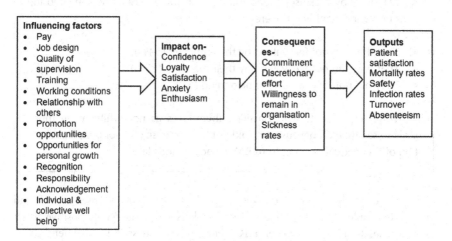

FIGURE 5.1 Factors affecting employee engagement.

along with appropriate education and training and support from their managers to fulfil their potential. It also places a duty on staff to take up the training offered to them. One of the *Our NHS People Promise* (NHS England, 2021) pledges is to support learning so that opportunities to learn and develop are 'plentiful', that all staff are supported to reach their potential and have equal access to opportunities.

The features of successful appraisals in the NHS (NHS Staff Council, 2010), have been summarised as:

- Both staff and managers take the process seriously. They prioritise it and prepare.
- Staff can clearly articulate the purpose of appraisals.
- Sufficient time is set aside for discussions.
- Actions and commitments are delivered.

Whilst the majority (but not all) NHS support staff have an annual appraisal, the evidence is that effectiveness varies. For NHS support workers appraisals and their associated development plans do not lead always lead to training or other developmental opportunities. In 2019, 86% of AHP support staff and 84% of nursing support workers reported in the (NHS England and Improvement, 2022) that they had an appraisal during the previous year. Whilst the majority agreed that it had made a positive difference to their work, a significant minority (29% and 26% respectively) reported that they did not think it helped them improve how they performed their job. Moreover, only a third of support workers reported that they had subsequently received any form of learning and development – other than statutory and mandatory, following it.

BOX 5.3 WHY DO PEOPLE QUIT JOBS?

A 2021 study by Mckinsey found that the top three reasons people cited for quitting their organisations were-

- That they did not feel valued by the employer (54%).
- That they did not feel valued by their manager (52%).
- They did not have a sense of belonging (51%).

Those respondents who classified themselves as non-white, were more likely to say that left because they did not have a sense of belonging – a reflection of the inequalities staff from BAME backgrounds face.

A small-scale study by Hyde and colleagues (2013), based on 60 interviews, found that NHS employees – including support workers – were generally positive about their appraisals, as well as other HR strategies such as staff involvement activities, team working and organisational communications. Staff perceived these as providing mutual benefits for themselves, their organisation and patients. As one support worker, quoted in the article, said: '[t]o give good patient care, you've got to have training, obviously ongoing training as well. And your appraisals come into that because when you have appraisals, you're discussing how you're doing your job, how you can improve, etc. Any way that you can improve obviously helps with patient care' (p. 304). Some interviewees, though, were less positive, seeing appraisals as something that was 'done to them' for the 'benefit of the organisation' (ibid., 301).

Griffin (2021) found that a quarter of mental health support workers had not had a development review discussion with their manager in the previous two years and, of those that had, only 36% felt that their appraisal had been 'useful'. Furthermore, less than half (40%) felt that their developmental needs had been subsequently met (ibid.). The same research discovered that 72% of respondents felt that they could perform more tasks if they were supported to do so. Kessler and colleagues' (2021 and 2022) survey of 4,000 nursing support staff employed in 148 NHS trusts found that a significant minority (21% of the sample) had not recently met with their manager to discuss their development needs, and of those that had over half (53%) reported that the training needs identified had not been met.

The evidence appears to be telling a consistent story. Most support workers do have an annual appraisal and are generally positive about the process. However, a significant minority do not have regular appraisals and for those that do, a large proportion report that the developmental needs they identify are not met.

There is little direct research on the process of appraisals in the NHS. Most of the studies that have been undertaken have investigated appraisals for General Practitioners. As we have just seen, what evidence there is suggests that support workers do not always feel that their appraisals are effective. It is not, though, clear why this is. Research on appraisals more generally suggests that one factor shaping their effectiveness is the extent to which appraisers, such as managers and supervisors, have confidence in their organisation's appraisal and development system themselves, as well as their organisation's workplace culture more generally (Brown and Lim, 2013). This may be a factor inhibiting the effectiveness of support worker appraisals. It may also be the case that appraisers are not always clear about what opportunities are available to support workers. Griffin (2021) found that mental health support workers felt that their managers would benefit from more training, information and support to help undertake appraisals. Furthermore, it may not be that appraisals are effectively run. Where they are and development opportunities are identified support workers may face barriers to accessing them, such as lack of funding (see below).

Making appraisals and development reviews work

Appraisals have multiple purposes. They are an opportunity for organisations to clarify their expectations of staff, to recognise those staff's efforts, to give them feedback, and to provide an assessment of performance (Brown and Lim, 2013). The appraisal process can involve subordinates or peers or supervisors – or all of them. Appraisals result in the setting of time limited (normally for a year) and specific goals, aims, tasks or activities linked to the appraisee's role. There is a body of research showing that the setting of achievable goals motivates people to act (Evans et al., 2020). Appraisals should also look ahead – identifying ways staff can develop in their current role or progress into a higher one.

Appraisals help employees to:

1. Understand their role.
2. Have an agreed set of priorities and objectives.
3. Identify and acquire the necessary knowledge, skills and behaviours to perform their role and meet their objectives.

Most NHS trusts should have written policies and support available for staff undertaking appraisals (this though is likely to be less so in primary care).

BOX 5.4 REFLECTIVE LEARNING AND LEARNING STYLES

One of the most widely used learning tools, which can support appraisals and development reviews, is David Kolb's Experiential Learning Cycle (ELC), although its use 'is often a matter of faith' rather than evidence (Tomkins and Ulus, 2016: 159). The ELC is based on the premise that learning occurs through experience, not just through information transfer. The longer you reflect on an experience, event, or action (which could be a task performed or an incident or an interaction with somebody else), the more likely it is that you will improve (Fee, 2011).

The ELC has four stages:

1. Concrete experience: The experience, event or action that is being reflected on.
2. Observation and reflection: This stage involves stepping back from the experience and reviewing it, which may involve asking the following questions: 'What happened?' and 'What was significant?'
3. Abstract conceptualisation: This comprises the process of interpreting the event and considering what would be done differently next time and what support, if any, might require enacting that change.
4. Active experimentation: This stage draws on the previous three and involves changing approaches to the experience. The cycle though does not end here. The modified action constitutes a new concrete experience which requires further observation and reflection.

Kolb did not just create the ELC, he also developed a partially linked Learning Style Inventory. Although it is unclear whether the Kolb intended each of the ELC stages to represent different learning styles or not (Bergsteiner et al., 2010), others have been more explicit, particularly Honey and Mumford (1982), who suggested the following styles are linked to ELC –

- Experience – Activist.
- Reflection – Reflector.
- Conceptualisation – Theorist.
- Experimenting – Pragmatist.

There are other attempts to categorise individual learning styles, such as Visual Learners or Physical Learner, the idea being if you understand your preferred way of learning (listening or through practice, for example) you can become a more effective learner.

Much of the research on learning styles, which is overwhelmingly based on university students, has focused on whether learning styles are stable. Is it the case that one person will be a reflector and another a pragmatist? Do we even all have preferred learning styles in the first place? Disappointingly the conclusion Bergsteiner and colleagues reach, in their review of the evidence, is that 'identifying differences in how individuals learn...is fraught with conceptual and empirical problems' (2010:30). Whilst the evidence suggests that care should be taken in assuming validity and reliability when considering styles of learning, the ELC does provide a useful way of thinking about development needs and can be of benefit to support workers.

Organising effective appraisals for support workers

What makes for an effective appraisal? From the start the point should be made that appraisals need to be part of an *on-going* relationship between the member of staff and their manager. On-going discussion and providing feedback, for example asking support staff about the training they have received or ensuring they can fully participate in team meetings, will mean that the appraiser is familiar with their support staff and their work. This will also mean it is not necessary for every achievement to be formally evidenced and that there are no surprises during the appraisal.

The following checklist is based on a review of NHS trust appraisal policies and guidance on best practice in respect of appraisals.

What do appraisers need to do?

1. The appraiser must prepare for the appraisal. This will include, except for new starters, consideration of the extent to which the appraisee has met the objectives set for them at their last appraisal, what has gone well and where there might be room for improvement along with potential future objectives. The

appraiser may wish to review the appraisee's job description and any evidence of achievement. This should be gathered during the year.

2. Appraisers should remind the appraisee to prepare for their appraisal in good time.

3. It should be ensured that there is sufficient time set aside for the discussion and that the appraisal takes place in a private space free from interruption. Appraisals normally take between one and one and a half hours to complete. Discussions should only ever be rescheduled if it is unavoidable.

4. The discussion needs to take place in an environment of openness and trust.

5. The appraiser should ask open questions, where possible, and maintain a genuine interest in the appraisee's answers and views. This requires the demonstrating of active listening.

6. The appraisee should do the majority of the talking during the appraisal.

7. Feedback should be constructive, with positives emphasised.

8. There should be no surprises. If there have been capability issues these should be dealt with as they occur not left to the appraisal discussion.

9. Appraisers should be aware of the development opportunities available and recognise that needs can be met in a wide range of ways, not just through formal learning.

10. Appraisers should support the appraisee throughout the year to meet their objectives including accessing any learning they might need. This may require some flexibility including amending objectives (with agreement) if circumstances change.

BOX 5.5 THE STRUCTURE OF THE APPRAISAL DISCUSSION

The NHS Staff Council (2010) suggested that the appraisal discussion should be organised as follows:

- The discussion should commence with a confirmation of the job content and requirements, followed by a general review of the last 12 months.
- There should then follow a more in-depth review of the previous objectives covering the appraisee's views of what has gone well, any concerns and issues and areas that may require further development.
- Next, clearly defined, and realistic objectives should be set for the following year.
- Personal Development Plans (PDPs) needs should then be considered, including the identification of future development requirements. (PDPs are discussed in more detail below.)
- The discussion should end with a summary of the talk, actions and plans.
- Following the appraisal there needs to be on-going discussions, feedback, coaching and reviews between the manager and member of staff.

What do appraisees need to do?

1. The appraisee should prepare for their appraisal, including thinking about their future aspirations and their organisation's values.
2. Where necessary, the appraisee should be able to demonstrate their achievements, and that they have completed learning (including statutory and mandatory training). Evidence of achievements might include a reflective diary, evidence of communications or commendations from service users or other staff, copies of presentations or course grades and evidence of attendance (Jackson and Thurgate, 2011)
3. Appraisees should play an active part in the appraisal discussion and be honest about their developmental needs.
4. Following the appraisal, appraisees should regularly refer to their objectives and development plan, taking the necessary steps to fulfil them (supported by their manager).

Effective Personal Development Plans (PDPs)

Based on the outcomes of an appraisal, PDPs identify, in a structured way, any learning and development needs that staff might have linked to their object-ives and practice. Developmental opportunities should take place before the next appraisal so as to support achievement of objectives, but also to allow the learning's effectiveness to be assessed. PDPs record progress (or barriers) to achieving devel-opment. They are the key output of the appraisal process, representing an ongoing formal agreement between the appraiser and appraisee. 'Having a PDP enables support workers to focus their workplace activities on achieving structured and achievable goals' (Jackson and Thurgate, 2011: 296). Development opportun-ities do not only mean accessing formal education. There are a wide range of other options that support staff can access to assist their development, including observing meetings, presenting, teaching, attending conferences, keeping a reflective diary, undertaking research, structured discussions with colleagues and coaching.

As we have seen a significant proportion of support workers who have had an appraisal report that the development needs identified in their PDP were not met. There may be a number of reasons for this:

- Lack of funding.
- Support workers are unable to take time off work.
- Lack of occupationally relevant learning available.
- Poor awareness of training that is available by managers and support staff.
- Lack of general career information and advice to help guide learning choices.
- Lack of buddies and mentors.
- Lack of opportunities to shadow or be seconded.

BOX 5.6 THE KNOWLEDGE AND SKILLS FRAMEWORK (KSF)

The KSF was developed as part of the *Agenda for Change* pay system in 2004. Its aim was to create a single comprehensive competency framework for all those NHS staff covered by the pay agreement, including support workers. It was intended to be used as part of the appraisal/PDP process to enable staff and their managers to identify, firstly the initial competences required to start working in a role (either on appointment or following promotion) and subsequently the competences required to become fully competent (as well as identifying developmental needs if they wished to progress beyond their grade).

At first the KSF contained 30 separate dimensions of skills and knowledge, each of which had numerous levels within them. However, the NHS Staff Council, (comprising trade unions, professional bodies and employer representatives), acknowledged that for some staff 'particularly in the lower bands, selecting the appropriate dimensions and levels and evidence to assess them has proved difficult' (2010: 14). Also employers did not exclusively use the KSF as the basis of assessing the competency needs of their staff. A study by the Institute of Employment Studies by Brown and colleagues (2010) for the NHS Staff Council found, in respect of the intended aims of the KSF, that whilst support for its principles were widespread 'the gap between the intended policy and the actual practice remains unacceptably wide' (p. ix). The study found that five years after its introduction, a third of NHS trusts did not use the KSF at all, and even where it was in use, it applied to only one in three staff.

In response, the NHS Staff Council proposed that employers focus on the six core dimensions of the KSF which are *Communications, Personal and People Development, Health, Safety and Security, Service Improvement, Quality* and *Equality and Diversity*. Guidance was also provided that sought to simplify the process (NHS Staff Councils, 2010).

There is no evidence available on whether the KSF is still being used by NHS trusts in England. Given its slow initial take-up and the lack of any further national 'push' to encourage employers to incorporate it into their appraisal processes, it is very likely that its use is very limited. I asked a number of senior NHS trade union and professional body officials whether they thought it was still being used, and they thought not. Intentionally or not the KSF's core dimensions do, however, appear in *The Care Certificate,* apprenticeship standards, along with support worker competency frameworks.

Whilst the focus of appraisals is mainly on the present – on how staff are currently performing their role, it is important that appraisals are also forward looking. A NHS trust in the Midlands, for example, as part of their appraisal process includes what they describe as 'talent conversations'. These allow staff, their supervisors and managers to consider future career aspirations and how those might be supported.

Equality, diversity and inclusion

'Our black and minority ethnic staff members are less well represented at senior levels, have measurably worse day to day experiences of life in NHS organisations, and have more obstacles to progressing in their careers.' (NHS England, 2021a: 3) Ensuring all NHS staff are treated fairly is not only a cornerstone of good patient care, but it also contributes to a more sustainable workforce and better organisational outcomes (Dawson, 2009; West et al., 2012; Kline, 2014; NHS England, 2021a; Jabbal et al., 2020; Hemmings et al., 2021). Unfortunately, the NHS's track record in this area, whilst improving, has not be great (Kline, 2014; Jabbal et al., 2020; Hemmings et al., 2021). It is the case, for example, that across 'an array of characteristics – including ethnicity, gender and religion – some groups are underrepresented in certain NHS careers' and efforts to address this underrepresentation have been 'limited' (Hemmings et al., 2021: 2). In fact, measures of equality, diversity and inclusion in the *NHS Staff Survey* have declined since 2015 (Jabbal et al., 2020).

Whilst almost one in five of support workers are from a BAME background, the numbers employed in individual trusts varies considerably from 68% of support workers at University College London NHS Foundation Trust to just 1.1% at Wirral University Teaching NHS Foundation Trust (NHS England, 2021b). We saw in Chapter 1 that support workers tend to be recruited from local labour markets. These labour markets reflect the diversity of local populations, which might explain some of the variation in the proportion of the support workforce from BAME backgrounds employed by NHS trusts (something to consider when planning *Outside/In* GYO approaches), although not all. The population of the Wirral comprises 5% of people from BAME backgrounds (Wirral Intelligence Service, 2019) for instance.

Data is gathered on the experience of working in the NHS of staff from BAME backgrounds through the *Workforce Race Equality Standard* (WRES), first introduced in 2015, and for those NHS staff with a disability through the *Workforce Disability Equality Standard* (WDES). The results of both provide insights into the lived experience of working in the NHS for such staff.

Whilst the data gathered from the WRES is not broken down by grade, it is very probable that BAME support workers relative experiences of working in the NHS are not dissimilar to BAME staff in registered grades. The data from the WRES (NHS England, 2021a) shows that whilst 21% of the NHS workforce are from a BAME background, they remain underrepresented in senior grades and on boards. Furthermore, BAME staff are less likely to be appointed to a job from a shortlist, than their white colleagues, and are slightly more likely to experience bullying, abuse or harassment from patients or the public (30% compared to 28%). BAME staff are also considerably more likely to report they have experienced discrimination from a manager. For AHPs, 13% of BAME staff reported discrimination compared to 5% of their white colleagues and 17% of BAME nursing staff did, compared to 6% of white staff.

Like the WRES, the gathering of WDES data is mandated and applies to all NHS trusts. WDES gathers data across ten metrics, including the proportion of staff in each pay band that has a disability, the proportion of successful applicants who have a disability and the percentage of disabled staff compared to non-disabled staff believing that the trust provides equal opportunities for career progression or promotion. Again, the data is not disaggregated so that it is possible to focus on the experiences of disabled staff in support worker roles.

In 2020, the proportion of the NHS workforce with a declared disability was 3.5% (NHS England, 2021c). The WDES (ibid.) reported on the experiences of people with a disability working in the NHS. It found that an NHS employee with a disability was 1.2 times less likely to be appointed to a new job from a short-list than a non-disabled colleague. Disabled staff were one and a half times more likely to be involved in a formal performance management capability process, than non-disabled colleagues. Over a quarter of NHS staff with a disability (26.3%), reported they had experienced harassment, bullying or abuse, compared to 18.5% of non-disabled NHS staff. More positively nearly eight out of ten (78.2%) believed they had an equal opportunity to progress their careers, although they did feel less valued than non-disabled staff (39% compared to 50%). Perhaps reflecting this, a quarter (26%) did not think that their employer had made reasonable adjustments to support them (House of Commons Library 2021)

Improving equality, diversity and inclusion: What works?

Potential HR interventions to improve inclusion include:

- Setting up staff networks for underrepresented groups in the workforce.
- Leadership programmes.
- Targets for representation at senior levels including boards.
- Career development programmes.
- Unconscious bias training.
- Allies.
- Reverse mentors.
- Creating opportunities for staff to safely raise concerns.
- Ensuring interview panels are diverse.
- Benchmarking data.

There is though a lack of substantial evidence on the effectiveness of such interventions in healthcare settings. Moreover, there are also likely to be 'no quick fix' or 'one-size fits all' solution (Jabbal et al., 2020: 10). For the NHS, Hemmings and colleagues (2021) suggest three conditions necessary to address equality and diversity which were that (1) there is sufficient data and information, (2) that there is an understanding of what works and (3) that there are sufficient resources and skills to implement and clear responsibilities for implementation. Jabbal and colleagues (2020) adds a fourth condition – leadership.

West and colleagues (2015), reviewed, in the context of the NHS, which HR strategies may be more successful in deliver improvements compared to others. They identify the following as particularly impactful:

1. Allies from non-disadvantaged/less discriminated against groups.
2. Providing training that leads to participants agreeing goals in respect of their own behaviours and attitudes in respect of equality and diversity. This was assessed as bring more effective than training that focuses on just informing people about unconscious bias, for example. Training about discrimination should include more covert forms, such as negative humour.
3. Asking people to take the perspective of a person who may be discriminated against.
4. Agreeing effective diversity policies, practices and procedures that include recruitment and selection, appraisals, disciplinary processes, job design, reward and promotion.
5. Coaching and mentoring of under-represented/discriminated groups.
6. The use of quotas to influence promotion decisions.

The WRES and WDES data seeks to provide benchmarks against which individual NHS trusts can judge themselves against. There is evidence that benchmarking can lead to some improvements (Jabbal et al., 2020).

Failure to create an inclusive work environment causes harm. Staff who are denied access to career progression opportunities or are ignored by senior staff or are excluded from networks of power, as nursing staff from BAME backgrounds can (Pendleton, 2017), experience 'physiological, psychological and behavioural consequences' (Jabbel et al., 2020: 6). Support workers, regardless of their ethnicity and/or whether they have a disability, already experience a number of barriers that can negatively impact on their careers. Whilst WRES and WDES data is not broken down by pay band, it is probable that the experience of support staff from underrepresented groups may be quantifiably worse still. Whilst progress is being made to make the NHS an inclusive place to work 'significant cultural challenges remain' (Jabbal et al., 2020: 22). This is underlined by a finding that improvements in WRES measures were linked to the extent to which organisations engaged with the equality agenda *prior* to the standards being introduced (Dawson et al., 2019).

Job design

Designing a job requires determining the roles and responsibilities of a position, how it relates to other roles and its place in the organisation's structure more generally (CIPD, 2019). Effective job design maximises employee's contribution to organisational objectives, as well as clarifying the knowledge, skills and behaviours required to perform that job, and ensuring staff have manageable workloads and rewarding work (ibid.).

Good job design matters in all organisations but given the nature of healthcare work and the importance, from a safety point of view, of ensuring that all patient-facing roles work within their scope of practice; job design in the NHS takes on an even more important function. As has been well rehearsed in this book, support worker roles have not been consistently and systematically designed. In maternity, for example, Griffin (2018) found no link between tasks performed and grading, and many researchers have recorded inconsistent allocation of tasks (see Kessler et al., 2021, 2022 for a further example). Amongst other consequences poor job design can inhibit delegation of tasks to support workers.

Inconsistent job design also means that the contribution of support workers to care is not always maximised. This is a significant issue when the NHS faces a shortage of staff. When working with the six maternity services in North West London to introduce a common band 3 job description, (see Box 5.7 below), discussions between them revealed differences in task allocations that had no basis in safe staffing, but rather existed because, as one midwife put it – 'we have always done it that way'. Working together to create one job description meant not only that MSWs across the area had a common roles and responsibilities, but also that capacity expanded as, following training, MSWs in one service started to perform tasks that they had not been able to before, but their colleagues in nearby services routinely undertook.

Attempts have been made in the past to address scope of practice for support staff, including guidelines for specific grades such as the RCM's (2011) *Roles and Responsibilities Guide for MSWs* guide. The later set out the tasks MSWs could and could not perform but did not distinguish between the responsibilities of different support worker grades. More recently and more substantially, education, competency and development frameworks have been developed that seek to define the boundaries of role, including between band 4 support roles and registered grades. These are discussed later. The next chapter will discuss the related issues of account-ability and delegation.

Formal learning opportunities for NHS support workers

The term 'formal learning' refers to any purposively organised education or training that leads to the acquisition of knowledge, skills and/or behaviours that are then transferred into practice. 'Training' is usually understood as learning linked to a work-related task or responsibility and 'education' as more general and broader learning. The two terms are, though, often used interchangeably and for the remainder of this section we will refer to 'learning' to encompass both. Formal learning may, or may not, result in a qualification. A foundation degree is an example of formal learning, but so is fire safety training or attending a conference or completing an on-line module on wound care. Learning in all its forms matters. Rafferty (1996) goes as far as to say that learning lies at the heart of nursing and there is good evidence for the benefits of learning for individuals, organisations and service–users.[1]

A key finding of all the research and reviews of NHS support workers is that they struggle to access occupationally relevant learning. As we have seen, this may be due to weaknesses in how appraisals are conducted or lack of understanding of what is available to support their development; however, support workers face further barriers when seeking learning. Before considering these and how to overcome them, the reasons why support workers want to learn – which they do – will be discussed.

What motivates support workers to learn?

Both Griffin (2021) and Kessler and colleagues (2021 and 2022) have explored the factors that motivate support workers to learn. The results are shown in Table 5.1 below. In Griffin's (ibid.) survey respondents were able to answer as many options as they thought applied to them, whereas Kessler and colleagues (ibid.), limited respondents to selecting just one motivating factor. In both cases, though, the main reason support staff wanted to learn was so they could either do their current job better or progress their careers.

Earlier Griffin (2018) explored, again through survey data, the reasons why MSWs engaged with learning. The reasons resonated with the findings in Table 5.1. MSWs wanted to access learning so as to develop new skills (89%), for personal development (80%), to increase confidence (54%) and for career progression (50%).

Barriers to learning

Whilst support workers are keen to access learning, they are not always able to do so. Kessler and colleagues (2021, 2022) survey of nursing support staff identified a significant number of barriers support staff faced. These are summarised in Table 5.2.

An investigation into the factors inhibiting the full development of support workers in diagnostic radiography services, identified the following learning-related barriers – the lack of available relevant education programmes, an absence of information about progression pathways, insufficient education capacity and a perception that support education is too complex (HEE, 2021a). In maternity the main barriers MSWs faced were – lack of funding (identified by 44%), lack

TABLE 5.1 Support worker motivation to learn

Reason for learning	Mental Health Support staff (Griffin, 2021) (%)	Nursing HCAs (Kessler et al., 2021) (%)
To do my job better	46	33
To progress my career	46	50
I enjoy learning	39	9
It was a requirement	16	6

TABLE 5.2 How significant are these barriers to your learning? (%)

Barrier	Extremely	Highly	Quite	Not at all	Don't know
Training is not on offer during work time	26.5	18.8	22.5	22.9	9.3
Not having English & maths	12.0	8.9	10.9	57.6	10.6
Lack of digital skills	9.8	11.9	23.5	43.0	11.9
Lack of support from manager	14.1	10.7	17.5	48.0	9.8
Not meeting entry requirements	16.3	14.4	18.1	34.0	17.2
Lack of confidence	15.0	16.5	25.7	36.3	6.5
Lack of knowledge about what is available	27.4	20.8	22.8	22.5	6.6
Lack of support from team members	14.3	12.1	18.3	46.8	8.6
The cost of training course	24.7	14.7	14.7	27.6	18.4
No personal return on my training (e.g. higher pay or career progression)	29.1	15.9	15.8	23.7	16.1
Desired qualification not available	18.2	12.0	15.1	33.7	21.1
Travel to college/training centre	11.2	10.0	16.0	46.7	16.0
Lack of flexibility in my role to balance work, home and study	22.5	16.3	19.3	29.5	12.4
Lack of (protected) study time	23.5	16.4	18.3	28.1	13.8
Lack of study skills	13.6	10.9	18.7	42.1	14.7

of opportunity (41%), workload (39%), time off (31%) and lack of management support (25%) according to Griffin's (2018) national survey. In a focus group one MSW summed up her situation which was common to many others – 'Time off for study leave is not supported, shifts aren't planned, its left to MSWs [to arrange cover for study]' (ibid., 33).

How can learning be improved for support workers?

Kessler and colleagues (2021, 2022), identified three enablers support workers who participated in their survey said would improve access to and completion of learning:

1. Support staff and their managers should be aware of the learning that is available.
2. Support staff need to be able and willing to participate in learning. This means ensuring they have protected study time and funding for example but also that issues such as self-efficacy are addressed. Self-efficacy is a malleable attitude

that refers to an individual's belief that they can deal with a situation or master a task or activity. Table 5.2 shows that a third of support workers feel that their lack of confidence is a barrier to learning. This also requires appropriate learning to be available, which is not always the case. The lack of appropriate courses was cited, for example, as the key reasons why radiography Assistant Practitioners were unable to progress their careers (Snaith et al., 2018).

3.   Support staff need to believe that the learning they undertake will make a difference.

Mental health support workers were asked to identify what steps could be taken in their view to improve their personal development, including learning opportunities (Griffin, 2021). These are shown in order of priority in Table 5.3.

NHS Education for Scotland (2019) interestingly asked support workers to highlight what features they thought characterised the design and delivery of good learning for them. They identified that learning should be:

- Fun.
- Engaging.
- Relaxed.
- Face-to-face.
- In small groups.
- Offer variety.
- A mixture of theory and practice.
- Structured.
- Interactive.
- Adapted to individual needs.

The support workers, who completed the NES (ibid.) survey also identified what that they believed needed to change to better support their learning at work. This was: a supportive learning culture (characterised by, for example, protected study time and more access to learning), with accurate information about how to progress their careers and learning that was relevant to their roles.

TABLE 5.3 Improving support worker development

Intervention
1. More effective appraisals
2. Transferable learning
3. Funding for training
4. Time off for training
5. Greater support for managers
6. Clear role guidance
7. Support to access pre-registration degrees
8. More training opportunities
9. Better guidance on training

The most significant development in VET in recent years has been the reforms of the apprenticeship system. This is true for the NHS, where a growing number of apprenticeships are available to support workers. These are designed to develop work-relevant knowledge, skills and behaviours, and, significantly, progression pathways.

Apprenticeships – the new gold standard or the only show in town for NHS support workers?

Apprenticeships are a form of work-based learning, designed to provide the apprentice with the knowledge, skills and behaviours they require for a specific job. This is achieved through a combination of experiential learning at work and off-the-job education. Apprenticeships are founded on a simple premise – that the best way to learn the competences needed for a job is through undertaking that job (Hager, 2013). As a result, apprentices are employees rather than students. Apprenticeships have a long history in the UK dating back, at least, to the medieval craft guilds in England. The first specific legislation concerned with them appeared in 1563. Since then, interest in apprenticeship by governments and employers alike has ebbed and flowed (House of Commons Library, 2015).

The most recent chapter in the history of apprenticeships began with an independent review of the system in 2012. This review (Richard, 2012) called for apprenticeships to be redesigned with a greater emphasis on outcomes, with more employer input and a recognition of industry standards. The review also called for all apprentices to reach a good level of English and maths and for incentives to be created to increase their take up. This led to an overhaul of apprenticeship system in England; the main features of which form the basis of the current system which began to be introduced in 2017.

The apprenticeship system

The apprenticeship system has the following features:

- The content of apprenticeships is designed and reviewed by employers from the relevant sector or occupation in Trailblazer groups. The RQF level 3 *Senior Healthcare Support Worker* apprenticeship, for example, which is the main one many support workers will complete, was developed by a Trailblazer Group that included: a care provider, NHS trusts, professional bodies, HEE and a hospice. Trailblazer groups continue to meet once apprenticeships are designed.
- Apprenticeships last for a minimum of one year. They include a formal qualification and have functional skill requirements. Where employees do not possess the necessary level of functional skills on commencing the apprenticeship (normally level 2), these can be acquired as part of the apprenticeship training. Apprentices cannot complete an apprenticeship until they have acquired the necessary level of functional skills, however.

- Completion of an apprenticeship is based on what is described as an End Point Assessment (EPA). EPAs assess apprentices through a number of assessment methods including tests, interviews and projects to assess whether they have acquired the necessary knowledge and skills. EPAs are conducted by an approved third-party organisation. For some apprenticeships EPA takes place at the end of the learning, for others, such as degree apprentices, it is integrated into the learning and an on-going process.
- The balance between work-based and 'off-the-job' learning is fixed by government as are costs, including EPA, through nationally set funding bands.
- Off-the-job learning can take on variety or forms and formats including on-line learning and formal learning in the workplace, as well as an education provider's classroom. From August 2022 off the job training must be a minimum of six hours a week.
- Employers, including NHS trusts, with annual pay bills in excess of £3million, pay 0.5% of their pay bill through a government apprenticeship levy that can only be used to fund training and EPA costs. The levy cannot be used for staff costs such as backfill. Unspent levy can, though, be transferred from one employer to a next. NHS trusts, for example, have supported training in care homes by transferring their unspent levy, which would otherwise be retained by the Treasury.
- Education providers such as ITPs, colleges and universities, but also employers (some NHS trusts are registered to deliver apprenticeships to either their own staff or staff of other trusts), and EPA organisations, must be government approved.
- For smaller employers, such as general practices, government grants are available towards the cost of learning and levy-paying employers are able to transfer any unspent levy they have.
- Apprentices have to be aged 16 years old or over. There is no upper age limit. Apprentices must be paid at least the national minimum wage.
- Apprenticeships have to deliver 'significant' new learning. Employees who have acquired a formal qualification in their occupation in the recent past, such as a NVQ, may not be eligible to start an apprenticeships in the same area. However, if staff have only acquired *The Care Certificate* they will be eligible to study, even though most apprenticeships relevant to NHS support workers include *The Care Certificate*.

Since the introduction of the apprenticeship levy and associated apprenticeship standards in 2017 apprenticeships have become the most significant vehicle for formal work-based education in the UK. This includes the NHS where there are a growing number of apprenticeships of varying lengths relevant to clinical support staff, starting at RQF level 2, and including degree apprenticeships (discussed in Chapter 7). In 2021 there were a total of 154 apprenticeship standards relevant to clinical and non-clinical NHS staff, and 22,000 NHS staff had started an apprenticeship during that year.

BOX 5.7 THE REGISTER OF APPROVED APPRENTICESHIP TRAINING PROVIDERS (ROAATP)

Organisations are able to apply to receive government funding to deliver apprenticeships. In 2022 there were three levels of provider possible:

1. 'Main' providers able to deliver full apprenticeships for their own staff and the staff of other organisations, as well as acting as a sub-contractor to other training providers. Some NHS trusts have achieved Main provider status.
2. 'Employer Providers' able to deliver full apprenticeships but only to their own employees.
3. 'Supporting Providers' can enter into sub-contracting arrangements with Main or Employer Providers to deliver elements of the apprenticeship.

Apprenticeships deliver a number of benefits for employers, employees and indeed society more generally. The National Apprenticeship Service (2018) found that 78% of employers they surveyed believed apprenticeships improved productivity and 73% that it increased staff morale. Apprenticeships allow employers to meet skill needs, improve organisational productivity and support innovation. They provide employees with work-relevant knowledge and skills, improve job satisfaction and lead to higher levels of pay compared to employees who have not undertaken them. Apprenticeships can further support social mobility. Apprentices earn whilst learning meaning that they remove financial barriers that prevent some groups from accessing education, as well as meeting education gaps, including functional skills (National Audit Office, 2018, 2019; Griffin, 2020).

Apprenticeships offer the opportunity to address a number of long-standing issues for support workers. They present a career structure, including into pre-registration education – and beyond. It would be possible, for example, to join NHS employment at band 2, complete a RQF level 2 apprenticeship, such as the *Healthcare Support Worker* apprenticeship, and continue at each pay band to complete a relevant apprenticeship until you reached master's level (RQF level 7) completing the *Advanced Clinical Practitioner* apprenticeship. Someone wishing to become a registered physiotherapist, for example, could pursue the following apprenticeship pathway:

- Health Care Support Worker Apprenticeship (RQF level 2).
- Senior Health Care Support Worker Apprenticeship (RQF level 3).
- Assistant Practitioner (Health) Apprenticeship (RQF level 5).
- Physiotherapist (Degree) Apprenticeship (RQF level 6).

- Enhanced Clinical Practitioner Apprenticeship (RQF level 6).
- Advanced Clinical Practitioner Apprenticeship (RQF level 7).

The content of an apprenticeship is determined nationally and includes formal qualifications, which should help address standardisation and transferability of learning for support workers. Whilst unquestionably a significant development for support workers, the substantial focus on apprenticeships and perennial lack of funding for other sorts of learning mean that there is a risk that apprenticeships become the only option available to support workers. This will be limiting. In any role, employees will only need to complete an apprenticeship once. Like registered staff, support workers need continuing professional development and more general supportive learning cultures as we will discuss.

Apprenticeships and the NHS

The NHS, as the country's largest employer, pays around £200 million into the apprenticeship levy fund each year. In a survey to all NHS trusts, with a 54% response rate, Unison (2019) discovered that almost 80% of trust's apprenticeship levy funds had not been allocated. A survey by Kessler, Griffin and Bach in 2019, exploring the approaches adopted by the public sector, including the NHS, to apprenticeships, found that three quarters of NHS trusts reported they would be unable to spend all their apprenticeship levy in 2019–2020. Two years later though HEE reported that 80% of NHS trust apprenticeship levy had been spent, including £13 million being transferred to other employers.[2]

Kessler, Griffin and Bach (2019) explored the motivation of NHS trusts for introducing apprenticeships and found that NHS employers saw them as a way of attracting new recruits (particularly younger employees) and as a means of upskilling existing staff – indeed most of the apprentices employed by the NHS trusts Kessler and his colleagues surveyed were existing employees not new starters. Half the NHS trusts surveyed had formal structures to oversee the delivery of apprenticeships and most (three-quarters) aligned their use with the trust's wider workforce strategy. There were limited examples of local trade union representatives being involved in NHS trust strategies and, at the time, the most frequently used apprenticeship standard was the Nursing Associate one (see Chapter 7). The survey also sought the views of employers on the barriers they faced when seeking to maximise the benefits of apprenticeships. These are set out in Table 5.4. The top two are related to capacity within the organisation.

Kessler and colleagues' (2021, 2022) survey of nursing support worker's education and training, asked respondents if they had been offered the opportunity to start an apprenticeship and, if they had, whether they were satisfied with it or not. The results are shown in Table 5.5. These show a gap at each level between those support workers interested in undertaking an apprenticeship and those offered the opportunity to complete one. They also show, for this group of support workers at

TABLE 5.4 Barriers faced by NHS trusts seeking to maximise benefits of apprenticeships

1. Lack of funds to cover backfill when staff are carrying out off the job training
2. Lack of capacity for mentors and supervisors to support apprentices
3. No funding available to pay the wages of apprentices
4. Concerns about the provision of quality education
5. Problems with arranging End Point Assessment

TABLE 5.5 Take up of apprenticeships by nursing support workers

Apprenticeship	Interested in	Offered	Not offered	Offered satisfied	Offered not satisfied
Healthcare Support Worker	34	25	75	90	10
Senior Healthcare Support Worker	43	20	80	83	17
Nursing Associate/Assistant Practitioner	59	17	83	66	32
Nurse Degree	55	14	85	67	32

least, a greater interest in the higher-level apprenticeship standards. The authors note this finding may be due to the fact that a very high proportion of the respondents (75%) wished to progress into pre-registration. Interestingly the survey shows high satisfaction levels for the RQF level 2 and 3 apprenticeships, but that this drops for the RQF level 5 and 6 ones.

BOX 5.8 EQUALITY AND TRAINING

There is a responsibility placed on employers by the Equality Act 2010 to ensure that training does not disadvantage any protected groups. An example of discrimination would be organising training on a day that people of a particular faith cannot attend.

Despite the interest in apprenticeships amongst support workers it is not clear how many are able to access them. Table 5.6 suggests that the numbers may be comparatively low compared to demand. Amongst mental health support workers of take up of apprenticeships is low, with just 1.8% having accessed either an RQF level 2 or 3 apprenticeship – despite the RQF level 3 having a dedicated mental health pathway. A slightly higher proportion (2.7%) had or were studying the Nursing Associate or Degree Apprenticeship apprenticeships (Griffin, 2021).

There is some limited evidence of the factors that might enable the successful delivery of apprenticeships in healthcare settings. Baker (2019a, 2019b), reviewing the literature, identified the following factors – appropriate levels of pay, clear information about the programme and appropriately designed roles as potentially underpinning successful delivery. McKnight and colleagues (2019) additionally pointed to the importance of partnership working between employers and education providers. On pay, Unison (2019) found variable approaches with 30% of NHS trusts paying the statutory minimum rate (and some even less than that). A review of NHS trusts in London also found a wide range of approaches to apprenticeship pay including paying of the minimum rate, spot pay and application of Annex 21 of *Agenda for Change* (Alma Economics, 2020).

BOX 5.9 CO-DESIGN AND DELIVERY OF APPRENTICESHIPS

Apprenticeships at RQF levels 2 and 3 for support workers will most likely be delivered by colleges or ITPs. Unlike universities, who are likely to deliver RQF level 4 and 5 apprenticeships (and above), these providers may not employ teaching staff with clinical experience. One solution to this is for the apprenticeship to be delivered in partnership with employers. This is what we did in North West London between 2019 and 2021, when the *Senior Healthcare Support Worker (SHCSW)* apprenticeship was introduced for the area's MSWs. The four West London NHS trusts with maternity services came together to jointly deliver, with an ITP. None of the NHS trusts were a Main provider, one was, though, a Supporting provider, one an Employer provider (see Box 5.7 above), and one was not registered on ROAATP. The *SHCSW* apprenticeship includes a specific maternity pathway. The ITP did not employ any midwives amongst its teaching staff. As a result, it was agreed that the ITP would support those learners who needed to acquire functional skills, as well as organise the learning administration, deliver core modules that were not maternity-specific and arrange the EPA organisation. Working together, the four NHS trust's Practice Development Midwives (PDMs) delivered the clinical element of the apprenticeship, drawing on the additional expertise of specialist colleagues when needed. The PDMs also worked closely with the ITP to ensure that the general content they delivered was contextualised to maternity. The PDMs calculated how much time they spent planning and teaching their elements of the apprenticeship. This included travel time, preparation, teaching (most of which was on-line due to the restrictions of Covid-19) and the time taken to assess learning. The PDMs also worked with the ITP to recruit the MSWs, making sure, for instance, that they possessed eligible qualifications. Based on the PDMs contribution, a proportion of the Apprenticeship Levy (the total cost of the apprenticeship, at that time, was £5,000 per apprentice) was returned to the NHS trusts. The NHS trust that was not on the ROAATP, had to second their PDM (for the proportion of time

> she spent delivering the apprenticeship) to the one that was registered as a Supporting provider.
>
> An (unpublished) evaluation of the apprenticeship found that the MSWs who completed it where positive about the learning experience and able to articulate the value of the learning. One reported: 'This training is designed to develop the MSWs. It is practically useful, and it is work based. It helps to enforce the understanding roles and responsibilities of MSWs and service standards which in turns helps us develop and provide better services.' Another explained clearly the effect she thought the learning had on care and safety: 'In terms of baby observation, before we had little or no knowledge on the subject which made us vulnerable to miss any critical signs of deterioration of the baby but now we know the vital signs to look for when observing and can report back effectively to the midwife when needed.'

A simulated cost-benefit evaluation of the RQF level 3 *Senior Healthcare Support Worker* apprenticeship within NHS maternity services in North Lest London (see Box 5.9) suggested a 'best case' return on investment to employers over six years of £60,088 per employee and a 'worse case' return scenario of £8,196 per employee. The same study interviewed senior midwives in the area implementing the apprenticeship about their *perceived* benefits, which they identified as:

- Releasing time for registered midwives.
- Improved safety.
- Improved functional skills.
- A more diverse and inclusive workforce.
- Service improvements such as increased rates of breast feeding, smoking cessation, vaccinations and improved observations.
- Reduced turnover due to a more satisfied maternity support workforce.

Other learning

Statutory and mandatory training

Like other NHS staff, support workers are required to complete workplace training that is required by law (called statutory training) to ensure a safe and healthy workplace, for example so that they have an understanding of the requirements of the *Health and Safety at Work Act 1974*, manual handling, risk assessment and awareness of the control of hazardous substances training. In addition, to statutory training individual employers specify mandatory training that staff must also complete. Such training, which might comprise, for instance, child protection, clinical record keeping, equality awareness, infection prevention and control, and resuscitation, is judged by organisations to be necessary for the safe and effective delivery of services, for example by meeting the national NHS standards for risk management or the standards of the Care Quality Commission (RCN, 2021). Such training should be paid for by employers and, wherever possible, take place in work time. New employees would be expected to complete their first statutory and mandatory (sometimes called together 'essential' or 'compulsory') training by the end of their first year of employment.

The Roadmap – *other learning programmes*

In 2022, as part of the *HCSW2020* campaign, NHS England sought to bring together in a *Roadmap* all the national learning programmes available to nursing support workers. Such a list will shift and change overtime but nonetheless offers an insight into what is available. It should also be said that the rationale for producing the *Roadmap* was an understanding that support staff were not clear about the opportunities available to them. The original list included a range of courses aimed at improving functional skills including programmes run by National Numeracy and Open Learn, as well as government schemes.

BOX 5.10 EDWARD JENNER LEADERSHIP PROGRAMME

The Edward Jenner programme, run by the NHS Leadership Academy, supports NHS staff, including support workers, to develop essential leadership skills and feel more able to deal with the daily challenges of working in healthcare. It leads to an *NHS Leadership Academy Award in Leadership Foundations* qualification. In an interview for this book, Gemma Hawtin, a Physiotherapy Assistant working in Leeds who attended the programme, told me: 'the Edward Jenner programme has given me the confidence to use my leadership skills. I now use what I have learnt as it enables me to empower the team I am with and the work we do with our patients. I had some [leadership] skills already without knowing'.

Other programmes and resources highlighted in the *Roadmap* included a free online resilience and wellbeing toolkit called *We Are Beyond,* information on coaching from the NHS leadership Academy (see also Box 5.10), and the over 400 online programmes provided by eLearning for Healthcare, which includes Autism Awareness and Communicating with Empathy, dementia awareness and support, wound care and end of life. Specific courses also exist for support workers employed in primary care (Primary Care Training, 2020) (www.primarycaretraining.co.uk/suitable-for/healthcare-assistants/).

BOX 5.11 *UNIONLEARN*

Established in 2006, *Unionlearn* supports unions in the delivery of on-line training opportunities for their members. The programme also supports *Union*

> *Learning Representatives* in workplaces (including in the NHS), one of whose objectives is to engage learners who might be hard to reach. Individual trade unions and professional bodies also have learning programmes available for their members including support workers.

In addition to the *Roadmap*, Skills for Health has developed a Skills Platform which seeks to bring together high-quality training programmes in a wide range of areas including supporting statutory and mandatory requirements, the learning elements of *The Care Certificate* and a large number of specific care and clinical programmes such as those teaching stroke awareness, wound care and immunisation and vaccination. Not all the courses on this platform are free, however.

The Higher Development Award

The Cavendish Review (2013) not only recommended the introduction of *The Care Certificate* for all health and social care patient-facing support staff, but also a common higher certificate. Despite the recommendation, this was not taken forward nationally. In North West London we recognised the demand from employers and support workers for a common programme that built on *The Care Certificate*, as Cavendish envisaged. One of the issues we were keen to address was building support worker confidence in learning and design training that could be delivered across health and social care for clinical and non-clinical roles. The programme, led by Dawn Grant, that was developed was called *The Higher Development Award* (HDA). Delivery of the HDA migrated to colleges, funded by the AEB not just in London but also other parts of the country. The HDA addresses study and functional skills and includes formal qualifications (a Level 1 pre-entry Endorsed award, a RQF level 2 Team Leader award and a RQF level 3 Leadership and Management award). With three levels, the programme supports a development pathway for learners. It also requires participants to deliver a service improvement programme. Fundamentally it aims to build learners confidence, self-belief and motivation. It also assists support staff access higher programmes: 'I have been able to complete the Care Certificate and then start and complete the Higher Development Award which enabled me to enrol onto the Trainee Nursing Associate apprenticeship.'

Dawn Grant told me that 'not everyone has a great experience at school, this can follow people into their working lives. In healthcare support workers get the job based on their caring ability, what we wanted to do was to support and recognise all their life experiences and build on this through personal development. The HDA has had a very positive affect on the daily lives of individuals who complete it, it improves their confidence, self esteem and knowledge base. It helps them to feel they fit in, feel part of the team, a parity of belonging. For those that need that level of development to remain in their role they feel fulfilled. For those wishing to progress their career it provides them with all the above plus the academic credit and focus to continue their career journey.'

NHS Support Worker Education, Competency and Development Frameworks

Along with the new apprenticeships, one of the other significant developments in respect of the deployment and development of NHS support workers has been the creation of national competency frameworks for specific occupational groups and conditions, such as mental health, radiography and cancer care. These seek to resolve the fundamental issues support staff have faced: lack of standardised entry-requirements, inconsistent job design (and therefore scope of practice) and truncated career pathways. Unfortunately, none of the frameworks are nationally mandated, meaning once again that their implementation is left to the discretion of individual employers and ICS's, however that is not to diminish their potential for support workers. We will consider two of the frameworks.

The Maternity Support Worker Competency, Education and Career Development Framework

Developed by the University of the West of England following a series of stakeholder events, and published in 2019, with the support of HEE, the *Maternity Support Worker Competency, Education and Career Development Framework* was the first attempt by the NHS in England to define the experience and education requirements and competences necessary for support staff. As we saw earlier the RCM (2011) had defined the tasks that MSWs could perform but not at each grade or the competences they required to perform those tasks or qualifications needed.

The MSW *Framework* has three career levels, each of which is based on Skills for Health's (2010) *Career Framework*. The first level in the *Framework* for MSWs (aligned with Skills for Health's level 2) is described as a Maternity Housekeeper role. This role undertakes 'basic care tasks' such as 'locating and filing notes, preparing documentation, general housekeeping...preparing women for clinical examination and tests, including screening and immunisation' (HEE, 2019: 10). This role does not however provide direct hands-on care.

The next level is described as a Maternity Support Worker. This role is aligned to Skills for Health's level 3. Maternity Support Workers 'may serve as a point of contact/support for women and their families and provide clinical, physical, psychological and emotional care and support' performing tasks such as routine maternal and neo natal observations, neonatal phlebotomy, infant feeding support and delivering parent education (ibid., 11). The final level, set at Skills for Health level 4, is also described as a Maternity Support Worker. This role is an extension of the previous one but additionally provides direct care 'acting as a point of contact for support or signposting' (ibid., 12) including to women and families that have more complex needs.

As well as defining role boundaries and career stages for MSWs, the *Framework* also sets out the competences staff at each of level require. These are placed within four domains:

1. Supporting women and families.
2. Public Health prevention and health promotion.
3. Personal and clinical skills.
4. Creating safe environments.

To take one example – within the second domain (Public Health) there are two competencies – *Promoting a culture of health and well-being* and *Actively engaging with public health initiatives*. Both of these competences are further broken down into a series of indicators. *Promoting a culture of health and well-being* comprises the following indicators:

- Influences on public health.
- Public health promotion.
- Making every contact count.
- Supporting behaviour change.
- Personal health and wellbeing.

Finally, within each of these indicators the details of what is expected of staff for each of the three roles is set out. Whilst some requirements are common across all roles, mostly there is a progression in complexity and demand. The MSW *Framework* also provides an indication of the expected qualifications (in terms of RQF levels) at each career level on entry and those expected to be acquired in-work.

The aim of the MSW *Framework* is to ensure mothers and families are supported by MSWs who are appropriately trained and have a clear scope of practice and for MSWs to have 'refreshed job descriptions and a more standardised career/development structure' (HEE, 2019: 4). HEE's Lead Midwife at the time, Sally Ashton-May, who led the development and implementation of the *Framework,* told me,

> the vital contribution maternity support workers make to the delivery of safe and personalised care for women and their babies is widely recognised. Our support workers are a valued, experienced, knowledgeable part of the maternity workforce with skills and competencies to safely and effectively support women, babies and families and be included as part of the midwifery workforce skill mix. Health Education England led the development of the Maternity Support Worker Competency, Education and Career Framework to provide a safe, robust and consistent approach to MSW education and training and supports the ongoing implementation in service.

There is evidence that the *Framework* is meeting that objective (Griffin, 2020). A MSW in North West London said,

> I think the framework is very clearly defined and easy to understand. The framework will help Maternity Support Workers to be more recognised and how important their work is for maternity and patient care. The far-reaching

recognition of Maternity Support Workers within and around the UK will allow their skills to be transferable between trust and different health care organisations which will be a great boost for the profession.

The Allied Health Professions' Support Worker Competency, Education and Career Development Framework

HEE adopted a similar approach to the MSW *Framework* for AHP support roles when it produced, with the support of AHP professional bodies and trade unions, the *Allied Health Professions' Support Worker Competency, Education and Career Development Framework* in 2021 (HEE, 2021b) – part of a wider strategy to increase the capacity and capability of AHP support staff. The AHP *Framework* seeks to be applicable to all the 14 AHP groups, as well as blended roles such as Therapy Assistants. The AHP *Framework* has a number of objectives for different stakeholders, including support workers:

- For ICSs, the AHP *Framework* seeks to support 'the standardisation of job descriptions and personal specifications across systems and networks and assess the relevance of current local training and education programmes, and work with employers and education providers to develop additional provision across the system' (HEE, 2021b: 6).
- For employers the aim is to work with others to support role and job description consistency and to 'review existing grade, skill mix and deployment to determine the need for new, extended, or enhanced support worker roles' (ibid., 6).
- For registered professionals and clinical staff, the *Framework* aims to ensure clear role boundaries, facilitate team working and better personal development plans.
- For education providers the aim is to 'support the design and delivery of occupationally specific education programmes, including apprenticeships' and enhance 'partnership working at system and individual employer level' (ibid., 6).
- For support workers the aim is help them to identify their developmental needs and professional and career development.

The AHP *Framework* is also based on three levels which are described as:

- *Entry level.*
- *Intermediate.*
- *Assistant Practitioner.*

Like the MSW *Framework* it also takes account of Skills for Health's (2010) *Career Framework*, although it additionally draws on a review of AHP job descriptions, formal education programmes, such as apprenticeships, existing professional body standards, research and input from AHP professional bodies. The AHP *Framework* sets standardised entry-requirements for each level. So, at *Assistant Practitioner* level new recruits are expected to already possess a RQF level 3 qualification (and therefore level 2 functional skills) and then acquire, over time, a RQF level 4 or 5 qualification such as a foundation degree, most likely through an apprenticeship.

Again, like the MSW *Framework* the AHP one has eight domains. In addition to *Formal knowledge and experience,* these are:

- Support patients and service users.
- Clinical, technical and scientific roles and responsibilities.
- Communications and information.
- Safe and inclusive environments.
- Research and service improvement.
- Leadership.
- Personal and professional values and behaviours.

Each of these domains are broken further down into individual competences with details of requirements set out for each stage.

Organisational learning cultures

So far, the focus of our discussion has been on formal learning. Over the years, though, there has been a shift in the way that learning is understood from being conceptualised as discrete 'packages' of knowledge and skills consumed away from the workplace in a classroom, to an understanding that it forms an integral part of work, supported (or hindered) by other processes and procedures such as coaching and appraisals (Fuller and Unwin, 2011). The everyday reality of work, as we saw in Chapter 2, is a continuous learning experience (for good or bad). Research suggests that the majority of what employees learn about their role may emerge from experiences such as feedback, observation, conversations, reading, attending meetings and listening (Griffin, 2013; HEE 2021c). Such learning is described as 'informal' or tacit learning. Unlike formal learning it is not planned or deliberate, indeed it is frequently accidental. The extent to which an NHS workplace might be described as a learning organisation, a concept first articulated by Peter Senge (1990)in his book *The Firth Discipline,* is important to the development and contribution of support staff (Kessler et al., 2020).

We discussed Fuller and Unwin's (2011) model of expansive-restrictive learning in Chapter 2. Their model presents a useful guide to assessing the extent to which support workers experience a supportive workplace culture of learning or not. In 2021 HEE (2021c) produced a guide to informal learning cultures, based on Fuller and Unwin (op. cit.) as part of its AHP support worker strategy. This proposed that employers audit their organisational culture by exploring the following (p. 5):

- The extent to which employees can draw on each other's experiences.
- Whether employees take a long-term view of their work and careers.

- Whether the learning and development of all staff is encouraged and is a key organisational objective.
- The degree to which learning, and development is spread across the whole organisation.
- Whether employees are encouraged to critically reflect.
- Whether managers are supported to assist their staff's learning and development.

Conclusion

Organisations that take a comprehensive approach to deliver 'good work' for their employees by implementing effective people-management practices have better outcomes, and healthier and happier employees (Ogbonnaya et al., 2017), including in the NHS (Ogbonnaya and Daniels, 2017). Good people management means the following (ibid.):

- Allowing staff to have influence over their work and a say in decisions that affect them.
- Jobs that are well designed with clear roles and responsibilities.
- An inclusive and supportive workplace environment, characterised by respect, good communications and team working.
- Staff receive fair and accurate feedback on their work and are supported by their managers and management processes.
- Staff have access to learning opportunities and are able to progress their careers.

Does this describe the experience of NHS support workers? In some, maybe a large number of services, probably but in others probably not. Whilst writing this book I talked to a clinical service head in an NHS trust, someone who is a real champion of the support workforce. Before she took up the role, her trust had celebrated that contribution of her service by, amongst other things, producing badges for staff to wear. But, she told me, these were not given to support staff, only to registered ones. It does not take much imagination to wonder how those support staff felt. One of the first things she did when she took up the role of service head was to make sure the support workers also had badges. She saw her workforce as one, her predecessor had not. The research evidence we have surveyed suggests, across all the areas, that constitute 'good work', the experience of NHS support staff can be poor, with consequences for the staff and for services. Many support workers experience a restrictive workplace learning environment. The good news, as we have also seen, is that all the elements needed to maximise the talent of support staff are in place. The even better news is that if they are mobilised then considerable positive outcomes will follow.

Checklist

- Effective people-management practices, such as appraisals, training and strategies aimed at ensuring an inclusive working environment, ensure not only that staff are able to thrive but also underpins high quality, safe and effective care. Staff who have a positive experience of work are more productive and tend to provide a positive experience for patients (amongst other benefits).

- Support workers do not always feel valued, or that they are full members of a team or able to access the training and development they need to provide the care and support they want too.
- NHS staff who have a disability or are from a BAME background are underrepresented in senior grades and are more likely to experience discrimination and harassment.
- The creation of occupational specific education, competency and development frameworks mark a significant development in the talent management of support staff.
- Assisting support workers to be the best that they can not only benefits them, but it will also benefit other staff, organisations and service users.

Notes

1 Research suggest well-organised learning can result in the following benefits: improvements in productivity, quality, reductions in innovation, supporting employees to cope with change, improvements in job satisfaction, higher wages and innovation (Griffin, 2013, chapter 3).
2 Communication from HEE with the author.

References

Alma Economics (2019). *Apprenticeships*. HEE (unpublished).

Armstrong, M. (2012). *Armstrong's Handbook of Human Resource Management Practice*, Kogan Page.

Baker, D. (2019a). Post-levy apprenticeships in the NHS – early finding *Higher Education and Workplace Learning*, 9(2), 189–199, 10.1108/HESWBL-10-2018-0114

Baker, D. (2019b) Potential implications of degree apprenticeships for healthcare education, *Higher Education and Workplace Learning* 9(1), 2–17 10.1108/HESWBL-01-2018-0006

Bellet, C., De Neve, J-E. and Ward, G. (2019). *Does Employee Happiness Have an Impact on Productivity?*, Saïd Business School WP 2019-13. Available at SSRN:https://ssrn.com/abstract=3470734 or http://dx.doi.org/10.2139/ssrn.3470734

Bergsteiner, C., Avery, G. C. and Neumann, R. (2010). Kolb's experiential learning model: critique from a modelling perspective, *Studies in Continuing Education* 32(1), 29–46. DOI: 10.1080/01580370903534355

Boornan, S. (2009). *NHS Health and Wellbeing*. London: Department of Health Available from: http://webarchive.nationalarchives.gov.uk/20130107105354/http:/www.dh.gov.uk/en/Publicationsandstatistics/Publications/PublicationsPolicyAndGuidance/DH_108 799

Bratton, C. and Gold, J. (2017). *Human Resource Management: Theory and Practice,* 6th Edition. Macmillan Education.

Brown, D., Mercer, M., Buchan, J., Miller, C., Cox, A. and Robinson, S. (2010). *Review of the NHS Knowledge and Skills Framework*. Institute of Employment Studies. www.employment-studies.co.uk/resource/review-nhs-knowledge-and-skills-framework

Brown, M. and Lim, V. S. (2013). Understanding performance management and appraisals: supervisor and employee perspectives. In Wilkinson, A., Redman, T. and Snell, S. (eds), *The Sage Handbook of Human Resource Management* (pp. 191–209), London, Sage.

Cavendish, C. (2013). *Cavendish Review. An Independent Enquiry into Healthcare Assistants and Support Workers in the NHS and Social Care Settings.* London, Department of Health. Available from: https://assets.publishing.service.gov.uk/government/uploads/system/uploads/attachment_data/file/236212/Cavendish_Review.pdf

CIPD (2021). Job Design. Available from: www.cipd.co.uk/knowledge/strategy/organisational-development/job-design-factsheet#gref

Clark, I. (2014). Healthcare assistants, aspirations, frustrations and job satisfaction in the workplace. *Industrial Relations Journal* 45(4), 300–313.

Dawson, J. (2009). *Does the Experience of Staff Working in the NHS Link to the Patient Experience of Care? An Analysis of Links between the 2007 Acute Trust Inpatient and NHS Staff Surveys,* July 2009, Institute for Health Services Effectiveness, Aston Business School.

Dawson, J., Sampson, J., Rimmer, M., Buckley Woods, H., West, M. and Nadeem, S. (2019). *Evaluation of the NHS Workforce Race Equality Standard (WRES)* NHS England. Available from: www.england.nhs.uk/publication/evaluation-of-the-nhs-workforce-race-equality-standard-wres (accessed on 6 February 2020).

Department of Health and Social Care (2021). The NHS Constitution. Available from: www.gov.uk/government/publications/the-nhs-constitution-for-england

Evans, M., Arnold, J. and Rothwell, A. (2020). *From Talent Management to Talent Liberation, A Practical Guide for Professionals, Managers and Leaders.* Routledge

Fee, K. (2011). *101 Learning and Development Tools. Essential Techniques for Creating, Delivering and Managing Effective Training.* London: Kogan Page.

Fuller, A. and Unwin, L. (2011). Workplace learning and the organisation. In Malloch, M., Cairns, L., Evans, K. and O'Connor, B. N., (eds), *The Sage Handbook of Learning.* London: Sage.

Griffin, R. (2013). *Complete Training Evaluation. The Comprehensive Guide to Measuring Return on Investment.* London: Kogan Page.

Griffin, R. (2018). *The Deployment, Education and Development of Maternity Support Workers in England. A Scoping Report to Health Education England.* RCM, available from: www.rcm.org.uk/media/2347/the-deployment-education-and-development-of-maternity-support-workers-in-england.pdf

Griffin, R. (2019). Maximising the contribution of Maternity Support Workers in North West London, *British Journal of Healthcare Assistants* 13(11), 149–151. https://doi.org/10.12968/bjha.2019.13.11.549

Griffin, R. (2020). *A Cost-Benefit Analysis of Enhancing Maternity Support Worker Roles through Utilisation of the Apprenticeship Standard to Implement the Health Education England Maternity Support Worker Competency, Education and Career Development Framework.* King's College London. Available from: https://healtheducationengland.sharepoint.com/Comms/Digital/Shared%20Documents/Forms/AllItems.aspx?id=%2FComms%2FDigital%2FShared%20Documents%2Fhee%2Enhs%2Euk%20documents%2FWebsite%20files%2FMaternity%2FMSW%20%2D%20Funding%2F04%2E%20MSW%20Evaluation%2Epdf&parent=%2FComms%2FDigital%2FShared%20Documents%2Fhee%2Enhs%2Euk%20documents%2FWebsite%20files%2FMaternity%2FMSW%20%2D%20Funding]

Griffin, R. (2021). *A Rewarding Job, but Frustrating Career. The Education, Development, and Deployment of Clinical Support Workers Employed in NHS Mental Health Services.* King's College London.

Hager, P. (2013). Theories of workplace learning. In Malloc, M., Cairns, L., Evans, K. and O'Connor, B. N. (2013) *The Sage Handbook of Workplace Learning* (pp. 17–31), Sage.

Health Foundation (2021). *Five Things We Learnt from Our Work on the Health and Wellbeing of Lower Paid NHS Staff.* Available from: www.health.org.uk/news-and-comment/newsletter-features/five-things-we-learnt-from-our-work-on-the-health-and-wellbe

HEE (2014). *Talent for Care. A National Strategic Framework to Develop the Healthcare Support Workforce.* Available from: www.hee.nhs.uk/sites/default/files/documents/TfC%20National%20Strategic%20Framework_0.pdf

HEE (2019). *Maternity Support Worker Competency, Education and Career Development Framework. Realising Potential to Deliver Confident, Capable Care for the Future.* Available from: www.hee.nhs.uk/our-work/maternity/maternity-support-workers

HEE (2021a). *Supporting Success. Developing Career Pathways for Diagnostic Imaging Support Worker Roles: Literature Review and Expert Group Survey.* Available from: www.hee.nhs.uk/sites/default/files/documents/DRad%20support%20workforce%20-%20literature%20review.pdf

HEE (2021b). *Allied Health Professions' Support Worker Competency, Education, and Career Development Framework. Realising Potential to Deliver Confident, Capable Care for the Future.* https://healtheducationengland.sharepoint.com/Comms/Digital/Shared%20Documents/Forms/AllItems.aspx?id=%2FComms%2FDigital%2FShared%20Documents%2Fhee%2Enhs%2Euk%20documents%2FWebsite%20files%2FAllied%20health%20professions%2FAHP%5FFramework%20Final%2Epdf&parent=%2FComms%2FDigital%2FShared%20Documents%2Fhee%2Enhs%2Euk%20documents%2FWebsite%20files%2FAllied%20health%20professions&p=true

HEE (2021c). *Making Learning Work for AHP Support Workers.* Available from: www.hee.nhs.uk/sites/default/files/documents/AHP_Guide_MakingLearningWork_Acc.pdf

Hemmings, N., Buckingham, H., Oung, L. and Palmer, W. (2021). *Attracting, Supporting and Retaining a Diverse NHS Workforce.* NHS Employers and The Nuffield Trust.

Honey, P. and Munford, A. (1982). *Manual of Learning Styles.* Maidenhead, Peter Honey Publications.

House of Commons Library (2015). *A Short History of Apprenticeships in England.* Available from: https://commonslibrary.parliament.uk/a-short-history-of-apprenticeships-in-england-from-medieval-craft-guilds-to-the-twenty-first-century).

House of Commons Library (2021). *Disabled People in Employment,* https://researchbriefings.files.parliament.uk/documents/CBP-7540/CBP-7540.pdf).

Hyde, P., Sparrow, P., Boaden, R. and Harris, C. (2013). High performance HRM: NHS employee perspectives. *Journal of Health Organization and Management* 27(3): 296–311. DOI 10.1108/JHOM-10-2012-0206

Jabbal, J., Chauhan, K., Maguire, D., Randhawa, M. and Dahir, S. (2020). *Workforce Race Inequalities and Inclusions in NHS Providers.* Kings Fund. www.kingsfund.org.uk/sites/default/files/2020-07/workforce-race-inequalities-inclusion-nhs-providers-july2020.pdf

Jackson, C. and Thurgate, C. (2011). Personal development plans and workplace learning. *British Journal of Healthcare Assistants* 5(6), 291–296.

Kessler, I. (2017). Exploring the relationship between human resource management and organizational performance in the healthcare sector. In Hitt, M.A., Jackson, S. E., Carmona, S., Bierman, L, Shalley, C. E and Wright, D. M. (eds), *The Oxford Handbook of Strategy Implementation.* New York: Oxford University Press.

Kessler, I., Griffin, R. and Bach, S. (2019). *Apprenticeships and the Pay Review Body Workforces: Final Report.* King's Business School. King's College London.

Kessler, I., Bach, S., Griffin, R. and Grimshaw, D. (2020). *Fair Care Work. A post Covid-19 Agenda for Integrated Employment Relations in Health and Social Care.* London: King's College London, available from: www.kcl.ac.uk/business/assets/pdf/fair-care-work.pdf

Kessler, I., Steils, N., Esser, A. and Grant, D. (2021). Understanding career development and progression from a healthcare support worker perspective Part 1. *British Journal of Healthcare Assistants* 15(11), 526–531, https://doi.org/10.12968/bjha.2021.15.11.526

Kessler, I., Steils, N., Esser, A. and Grant, D. (2022). Understanding career development and progression from a healthcare support worker perspective Part 2. *British Journal of Healthcare Assistants* 16(1), 6–10. https://doi.org/10.12968/bjha.2022.16.1.6

Kline, R. (2014). *The 'Snowy White Peaks' of the NHS: A Survey of Discrimination in Governance and Leadership and the Potential Impact on Patient Care.* Available from: Middlesex University www.england.nhs.uk/wp-content/uploads/2014/08/edc7-0514.pdf

Mckinsey (2021), *Great Attrition or Great Attraction? The Choice Is Yours.* Available from: www.mckinsey.com/business-functions/people-and-organizational-performance/our-insights/great-attrition-or-great-attraction-the-choice-is-yours

McKnight, S., Collins, S. L., Way, D. and Iannotti, P. (2019). Case study: establishing a social mobility pipeline to degree apprenticeships. *Higher Education, Skills and Work-Based Learning* 9(2), 149–163. https://doi.org/10.1108/HESWBL-01-2019-0012

National Audit Office (2018). *Achieving the Benefits of Apprenticeships. A Guide for Employers.* National Audit Office. Available from: https://assets.publishing.service.gov.uk/government/uploads/system/uploads/attachment_data/file/800060/Achieving_the_benefits_of_apprenticeships.pdf

National Apprenticeship Service. (2018). *Achieving the Benefits of Apprenticeships. A Guide for Employers.* National Apprenticeship Service. Available from: https://assets.publishing.service.gov.uk/government/uploads/system/uploads/attachment_data/file/800060/Achieving_the_benefits_of_apprenticeships.pdf

NHS Education for Scotland (2019). *Healthcare Support Worker Learning Survey, 2018.* NHS Education for Scotland. Available from: www.hcswtoolkit.nes.scot.nhs.uk/media/37982/nes1030_nes_hcsw_learning_survey_2018_final.pdf

NHS England (2019). *Interim People Plan.* Available from: www.longtermplan.nhs.uk/wp-content/uploads/2019/05/Interim-NHS-People-Plan_June2019.pdf

NHS England (2021a). *Workforce Race Equality Standard, 2020 Data Analysis Report for Trusts and Clinical Commissioning Groups.* Available from: www.england.nhs.uk/publication/workforce-race-equality-standard-2020-supporting-data/

NHS England (2021b). *Workforce Race Equality Standard 2020: Supporting Data.* Available from: www.england.nhs.uk/publication/workforce-race-equality-standard-2020-supporting-data/

NHS England (2021c). *Workforce Disability Equality Standard. 2020 Data Analysis for NHS Trusts and Foundation Trusts.* Available from: www.england.nhs.uk/wp-content/uploads/2021/10/wdes-2020-data-analysis-report.pdf

NHS England and NHS Improvement (2022). *NHS Staff Survey.* Survey Coordination Centre. Available from: www.nhsstaffsurveys.com

NHS Staff Council (2010). *Appraisals and KSF Made Simple – a Practical Guide. NHS Employers.* Available from: www.nhsemployers.org/sites/default/files/2021-07/Appraisals-and-KSF-made-simple.pdf

Nuffield Trust (2020). *Untapped? Understanding the Mental Health Clinical Support Workforce.* Nuffield Trust, available from: www.nuffieldtrust.org.uk/research/untapped-understanding-the-mental-health-clinical-support

Ogbonnaya, C., Daniels, K., Connolly, S. and van Veldhoven, M. (2017). Integrated and isolated impact of high performance work practices on employee health and well-being: A comparative study. *Journal of Occupational Health Psychology* 22, 98–114.

Pendleton, J. (2017). The experiences of black and minority ethnic nurses working in the UK. *British Journal of Nursing* 26(1), 37–42.

Rafferty, A. M. (1996). *The Politics of Nursing Knowledge.* Routledge.

RCM (2011). *The Role and Responsibilities of MSWs*. RCM. Available from: www.rcm.org.uk/media/2338/role-responsibilities-maternity-support-workers.pdf

RCN (2021). *Training: Statutory and Mandatory*. Available from: www.rcn.org.uk/get-help/rcn-advice/training-statutory-and-mandatory

Richard, D. (2012). *Richard Review of Apprenticeships*. Department for Business, Innovation and Skills. Available from: www.gov.uk/government/publications/the-richard-review-of-apprenticeships

Senge, P. (1990). *The Fifth Discipline: The Art and Practice of Learning Organisations*. London, Century Business.

Skills for Health (2010). *Key Elements of the Career Framework*. Available from: https://skillsforhealth.org.uk/wp-content/uploads/2020/11/Career_framework_key_elements.pdf

Tomkins, L. and Ulus, E. (2016). 'Oh, was that "experiential learning"?!' Spaces, synergies and surprises with Kolb's learning cycle. *Management Learning* 47(2), 158–178.

Unison (2019). The apprenticeship levy and the NHS: It does not add up. *British Journal of Healthcare Assistants* 13(11), 561–563.

West, M. A. and Dawson, J. F. (2012). *Employee Engagement and NHS Performance*. Kings Fund London. Available from: www.kingsfund.org.uk/sites/default/files/employee-engagement-nhs-performance-west-dawson-leadership-review2012-paper.pdf

West, M., Dawson, J. and Kaur, M. (2015). *Making the Difference. Diversity and inclusion in the NHS*. Kings Fund. Available from: www.kingsfund.org.uk/sites/default/files/field/field_publication_file/Making-the-difference-summary-Kings-Fund-Dec-2015.pdf

Wirral Intelligence Service (2019). *Wirral Population*. Available from: www.wirralintelligenceservice.org/state-of-the-borough/wirral-population/

6

REGULATION, DELEGATION AND SUPERVISION

Introduction

In 2014 after planning implementation of *The Care Certificate* in North West London, we decided to come together with colleagues from general practice and social care to launch the programme. The event was held in the rather lovely setting of the Grade 1 listed art deco Mary Ward Conference Centre in the heart of Bloomsbury. One of the speakers Loo Blackburn, a Practice Nurse by background, talked about the implementation of *The Care Certificate* in primary care and made the point that the person who cut her hair was subject to more regulation and training than health and social care support workers. Robert Francis (2013) made a similar point, when he pointed out that a taxi driver taking a patient to hospital has to meet more formal standards than support workers. He went on to say that there was almost no protection for the public because support workers lacked minimum standards of training or competence. He also made the point that support staff could be dismissed by one employer because they were judged as unfit to practice but there was no system that would allow a future employer to know this, meaning that they could potentially continue to work in the NHS. Consequently Francis recommended that support workers be regulated (see Box 6.1).

This chapter is about regulation, accountability, delegation and supervision. In the absence of formal registration of NHS clinical support staff, understanding of responsibilities and particularly ensuring that allocation of tasks to support staff (and their acceptance) is appropriate and supported is the cornerstone of safe care. Regulatory bodies such as the Nursing and Midwifery Council set standards for delegation and supervision and professional bodies provide further guidance; however, the inconsistent deployment of NHS support staff suggests that a range of factors may impact of individual decisions to delegate of not. We will consider what other factors may enable or inhibit task allocation.

DOI: 10.4324/9781003251620-12

Regulation

Regulation refers to the processes, standards and procedures designed to ensure that the actions, behaviours, values, skills and knowledge necessary to underpin safe, effective and compassionate care are in place. In the aftermath of the Francis Inquiry (2013) there was an expectation that his recommendation that patient-facing support workers should be regulated would be accepted, particularly as this was supported by professional bodies such as the RCN (based on the need for protect patients). One not untypical headline at the time was 'Support Workers face compulsory regulation on the back of Mid Staffs probe' (Community Care, 2013). The Health Select Committee concluded that the 'evidence is strongly in favour of at least a compulsory registration scheme, and the imposition of common standards of training and a code of conduct' (quoted in National Health Executive, 2013).

Whilst in the immediate aftermath of the Francis inquiry, the government briefly mooted the possibility of a voluntary register for support staff, both the NHS chief executive, Sir David Nicholson and the Chief Nursing Officer, Dame Christine Beasley, in their evidence to Francis, indicated their opposition to formal regulation. This was on the grounds that the costs of doing so were disproportionate in terms of patient safety (National Health Executive, 2013). As we saw in Chapter 2 the only changes actually implemented following the inquiry for support staff were a new code of conduct and *The Care Certificate*. This means that because 'a quarter of NHS staff are unregulated support workers, the majority of them nursing assistants' there continues to be a 'significant debate about whether such unregulated staff should be brought within a statutory regime' (Health Foundation, 2016: 15).

BOX 6.1 WHAT FORM OF REGULATION FOR SUPPORT WORKERS DID ROBERT FRANCIS RECOMMEND?

Francis proposed a minimalist approach to regulation based on a national register maintained by a regulatory body and unique identifiers for staff. The register would include the current and previous employers of support staff, their address, and any reasons, reported by their employer, as to why their previous employment ended. The support workers could record, if they wished, any views on the reasons for employment termination.

Whilst Nursing Associates (discussed in the next chapter) are regulated by the Nursing and Midwifery Council it does not seem that formal registration of support workforce as a role with regulatory bodies, such as the General Chiropractic Council, General Optical Council, Health and Care Professions Council, is likely any time soon. Registration is not, though, the only way to protect patients. In response to the Francis inquiry the government argued that *Disclosure and Barring Service* checks and *The Care Certificate* would help ensure protection, although the effectiveness of both has been questioned (Health Foundation, 2016). The creation of apprenticeship standards with national curriculums should help, over time, to standardise roles including their scope of practice, as will the competency frameworks and guidance from professional bodies, discussed in the previous chapter. In the absence of a national system of regulation, however, the extent to which any of these are effective depends on local decisions. As the Health Foundation (2016) has pointed out policy makers have placed the responsibility 'to ensure that unregulated staff are properly trained and conduct themselves appropriately' on employers and registered staff who delegate tasks to them (p. 23).

Accountability

Employers, registered staff and support workers are all legally accountable for the delivery of safe patient care. Employers are legally accountable for the actions of their employees (called vicarious liability) and must ensure sure have appropriate training and supervision. Staff have a responsibility to their employers and registered staff additionally to regulatory bodies, who set standards including for delegation of tasks (below). All healthcare staff, including support workers, have a duty of care in law to their patients and a legal liability in respect of the tasks they perform (Nursing and Midwifery Council, 2020a; RCN, 2022).

Delegation

Delegation refers to the transfer of tasks, responsibilities or authority from one individual to another. This could be between registered staff from the same or different professions, from a registered member of staff to a support worker or another person such as a Personal Assistant. Delegation can take a number of forms –direction, guidance, observation, joint working, discussion, exchange of ideas and co-ordination of activities (Chartered Society of Physiotherapy, 2020). It can be in person, or under the right circumstances such as with qualified mammography associates in a mobile screening unit, virtual. The setting in which delegation and supervision takes place, for example in a hospital department or community setting, always needs to be taken into account when deciding which tasks to delegate.

All those involved in delegation, including employers, have responsibilities and obligations to ensure that it is safe. The Nursing and Midwifery Council's (2020b) *The Code – Professional standards of practice and behaviour for nurses, midwives and nursing associates* sets out guidance for registered staff considering the delegation of tasks. Code 11 states that they are accountable for their decisions to delegate and that they should only delegate tasks and responsibilities that are within the other person's scope of competence, making sure that the other employee has fully understood any instructions. The Nursing and Midwifery Council further places a duty on registered staff to ensure that there is adequate supervision and support to 'provide safe and compassionate care' and that the outcome of delegation 'meets the required standard' (p. 12). *The Code* (ibid.) contains 24 standards, all of which apply to Nursing Associates as a registered role.

BOX 6.2 RCN PRINCIPLES OF DELEGATION TO SUPPORT WORKERS

- Delegation must always be in the best interest of the patient and not performed simply to save time or money.
- The support worker must have been suitably trained to perform the intervention.
- Full records of training, including dates, should be kept.
- Evidence that the support workers' competence has been assessed should be recorded, preferably against recognised standards.
- There should be clear guidelines and protocols in place so that the support worker is not required to make a standalone clinical judgement.
- The delegated task or responsibility should be within the support worker's job description.
- The team need to be informed that the activity has been delegated.
- The person who delegates the task must ensure that an appropriate level of supervision is available and that the support worker has the opportunity for mentorship. The level of supervision and feedback needed depends on the recorded knowledge and competence of the support worker, the needs of the patient/client, the service setting and the activities assigned.
- Support workers must have ongoing development to make sure their competency is maintained.
- The whole process must be assessed to identify any risks.
- The support worker then carries the responsibility for that task.

(Source: RCN, 2022)

The Health and Care Professions Council, which regulates AHPs, has similar standards to the Nursing and Midwifery Council in respect of delegation. Standard 4 (Health and Care Professions Council, 2018a) states that tasks should only be delegated to someone with the knowledge, skills and experience to carry out that work and that they should receive appropriate support and supervision. The Chartered Society of Physiotherapy (2020) provides its members with extensive advice on the factors that should underpin decisions whether tasks and duties should be delegated or not by a registered physiotherapist to a physiotherapy support worker. These include the responsibilities of support workers (pp. 3–4):

- 'The primary motivation for delegation is to serve the interests of the patient/ client.
- The registered practitioner undertakes appropriate assessment, planning, implementation and evaluation of the delegated role.

- The person to whom the task is delegated must have the appropriate role, level of experience and competence to carry it out.
- Registered practitioners must not delegate tasks and responsibilities to colleagues that are beyond their level of skill and experience.
- The support worker should undertake training to ensure competency in carrying out any tasks required. This training should be provided by the employer.
- The task to be delegated is discussed and if both the practitioner and support worker feel confident, the support worker can then carry out the delegated work/task.
- The level of supervision and feedback provided is appropriate to the task being delegated. This will be based on the recorded knowledge and competence of the support worker, the needs of the patient/client, the service setting and the tasks assigned.
- Regular supervision time is agreed and adhered to.
- In multi-professional settings, supervision arrangements will vary and depend on the number of disciplines in the team and the line management structures of the registered practitioners.
- The organisational structure has well defined lines of accountability and support workers are clear about their own accountability.
- The support worker shares responsibility for raising any issues in supervision and may initiate discussion or request additional information and/or support.
- The support worker will be expected to make decisions within the context of a set of goals /care plan which have been negotiated with the patient/client and the health care team.
- The support worker must be aware of the extent of his/her expertise at all times and seek support from available sources, when appropriate.
- Documentation is complete.'

Despite the clarity of such guidance, the evidence we are now familiar with is that the distribution of tasks and responsibilities between registered professionals and support staff in the NHS is not even, across occupations or within individual settings. This can lead to staff being underutilised – not being delegated tasks that they could safely perform (Richards, 2020; Griffin, 2021; Kessler et al., 2021, 2022) or on occasions being asked to perform tasks beyond their scope of practice or level of training (Griffin, 2018).

The absence of detailed guidance in many areas about what duties support workers can and cannot perform no doubt is a significant contributor to this incon-sistency. This, for example, led to the development of essentially lists of tasks that support workers in maternity (RCM, 2011) and diagnostic radiography (HEE, 2021a) can undertake. What else, though, shapes the decision of registered staff to delegate a task or not? Kessler, Heron and Dopson (2015) explored the issue of why registered staff decide to delegate or not through the lens of the broader research on professionalization – defined by them as moves by professionals, such as nurses, doctors, and teachers, to claim sole jurisdiction over certain work activities. They note, in a review of the literature, that the rise of the HCA role in the 1990s (discussed in Chapter 1) led some nurses to *discard* routine tasks but others to *hoard* them. They found that there were tasks register staff could have safely delegated but that they did not. The reason for this was that some nurses saw the importance of the profession being holistic, i.e., engaged in *all* the duties that nursing embraced. Support workers for these staff were seen as a threat by encroaching on that holistic vision of work. Kessler and colleagues (ibid.) make the point that the nursing profession is characterised by a 'divided self' – on the one hand articulating the logic of discarding tasks but on the other also of hoarding. Support staff potentially operate within this contested space.

BOX 6.3 RCM DELEGATION GUIDANCE

The RCM's (2011) *Role and Responsibilities of Maternity Support Workers* has the following guidance in respect of delegation:

- 'The decision whether or not to delegate a task should be made solely by a midwife based on their clinical judgement. The midwife is responsible and accountable for any decision to delegate.
- MSW role boundaries should be clearly and unambiguously defined and reflected in up-to-date job descriptions and person specifications.
- All staff are made aware of the tasks that MSWs can and cannot perform.
- Delegation should be the responsibility of a single midwife to avoid confusion, omission or duplication.' (p. 8)

Exploring, in a hospital setting, the attitudes of nurses and support staff, Kessler and his fellow authors, found examples of both sides of the profession's 'divided self'. Most nurses were positive about support workers, with a typical comment being 'nurses recognize they couldn't do their job if they didn't have the support of the HCAs' (p. 745). There were, though, a minority who perceived support staff as a threat to their holistic model of nursing, with one saying, for example, that 'health care assistants do a lot of the hands-on care. It sort of goes against the grain for me because I was trained when actually the nurse did all the hands-on care' (p. 746). Kessler and colleagues also noted that nurse's confidence in individual support workers was shaped by their perception of the support workers experience, capability, and orientation to their role. The study concluded that 'our findings are largely consistent with the assumptions underpinning a specialist–discard logic: The HCA relieves the nurse of the "burdensome" or "dangerous" routine tasks allowing them to concentrate on more technically advanced tasks and, in so doing, advancing their professional project.' (p. 748)

Daykin and Clarke's (2000) research, discussed in Chapter 1, echoes the finding that although many nurses saw the importance of their role being holistic, they were quite content to delegate certain tasks, those associated with 'dirty work' to support staff. The extent to which registered staff are hoarders or discarders is likely to some degree to shape delegation decisions. Potter and colleagues (2010) described how conflict often characterised delegation, with effective delegation occurring when there were good working relations, communication and teamwork. Tardivel (2012) also found delegation could be 'contentious' in part due to ambiguous role design. Pringle (2017) investigated the delegation of urinary catheterisation to nursing community support workers and found some reluctance by registered staff to delegate, again due to a lack of clear national guidelines. She also felt that education should be provided to the district nurses to give them more confidence to delegate.

This discussion suggests that the decision to delegate a task or not may be shaped by more than just processes and procedures, although lack of clear guidance inhibits delegation.[1]

Professor Kessler and I planned to investigate the factors that might shape a registered professional's propensity to delegate (nor not) to a support worker. We developed a model that suggested this was potentially influenced by the member of staff's background (age, experience, grade, training and area of work for example), their professional identity, role clarity, risk aversion, perceptions of accountability, and trust in the person they are delegating too. Unfortunately, we did not get the opportunity to test this model out in the field, but an investigation of the factors leading to decisions to delegate medication management in community settings from registered to unregistered staff, by Shore and colleagues (2022), did identify multiple factors influencing decisions. These comprised national guidance (which, when not clear, inhibited delegation), organisational factors such as communications and the presence of champions, as well as the relationship between staff. Relationships were influenced by personal views and possession of occupationally relevant education. This points to delegation being a multifaceted concept and may explain why support workers are not always able to perform tasks they are competent too (along with poor job design and restricted access to education).

Supervision

The AHP support worker competency framework (HEE, 2021b) discussed in the last chapter, makes clear that 'until support workers can demonstrate that they are able to perform tasks and responsibilities competently and safely for each stage [of the framework] they should be closely supervised by an appropriately qualified and registered member of staff' (p. 9). All the guidance on delegation discussed above stresses the need for an appropriate level of supervision, along with other support such as mentorship and feedback. The degree of supervision provided will depend on the formal knowledge and competence of the support worker, the needs of patients, location of work and task allocated Points to consider in respect of supervision are –

- Staff can only supervise within their own scope of practice.
- If the member of staff supervising is from a different profession from the support worker, they should seek advice and guidance from a more senior member of staff in the support worker's profession. An example might be a registered nurse delegating tasks to a MSW on a post-natal ward.
- Time should be set aside for the supervisor and supervisee to discuss and record.
- Support staff should raise any concerns that they might have, including whether they think that they are receiving sufficient supervision and support.
- Provision should be made for someone else to act in the role of supervisor, when that member of staff is absent, for example when they are on leave.

Supervision is a key element of safety, but it is not just about management. The Health and Care Professions Council (2018b) point out the effective supervision helps solves problems, supports professional development, improves the quality of care and practice.

Conclusion

Appropriate delegation and effective supervision underpin safe care. Getting this right also though improved patient outcomes. A systematic review by Snowdon and colleagues (2020) found evidence that delegation by AHPs to therapy assistants led to reduced length of stays (when assistants supervised exercises in a hospital setting) and reduced mortality after hip fracture, when assistants provide nutritional and feeding support to patients. Appropriate delegation, reflecting the needs of service users, frees up the time of busy registered staff. Decisions to delegate despite considerable information and guidance varies within and between workplaces and professions. A number of factors may shape this including professional identity, risk aversion and the support workers access to occupationally relevant education.

Note

1 I was told that the RCM's (2011) guide on tasks that MSWs could perform was their most downloaded publication, suggesting the degree of need form registered and unregistered staff.

References

Chartered Society of Physiotherapy. (2020). Information Paper. Supervision, Accountability and Delegation. Available from: www.csp.org.uk/publications/supervision-accountability-delegation-activities-support-workers-guide-registered

Community Care (2013). Support workers face compulsory regulation on the back of Mid Staffs probe. Available from: www.communitycare.co.uk/2013/02/06/support-workers-face-compulsory-regulation-on-back-of-mid-staffs-probe/

Daykin, N. and Clarke, B. (2000). 'They'll still get the bodily care'. Discourses of care and relationships between nurses and health care assistants in the NHS. *Sociology of Health & Illness* 22(3), 349 –363.

Francis, R. (2013). *Report of the Mid Staffordshire NHS Foundation Trust Public Health Inquiry.* Available from: www.gov.uk/government/publications/report-of-the-mid-staffordshire-nhs-foundation-trust-public-inquiry

Griffin, R. (2018). *The Deployment, Education and Development of Maternity Support Workers in England. A Scoping Report to Health Education England. RCM.* Available from: www.rcm. org.uk/media/2347/the-deployment-education-and-development-of-maternity-support-workers-in-england.pdf

Griffin, R. (2021). *A Rewarding Job, But Frustrating Career. The Education, Development, and Deployment of Clinical Support Workers Employed in NHS Mental Health Services.* King's College London

The Health Care Professions Council (2018a). *Standards of Conduct, Performance and Ethics.* Available from: www.hcpc-uk.org/standards/standards-of-conduct-performance-and-ethics/

The Health Care Professions Council (2018b). *Supervision and Delegation.* Available from: www.hcpc-uk.org/covid-19/advice/applying-our-standards/supervision-and-delegation/

Health Foundation (2016). *Fit for Purpose? Workforce Policy in the English NHS.* Available from: www.health.org.uk/publications/fit-for-purpose

HEE (2021a). *Supporting Success Developing Career Pathways for Diagnostic Imaging Support Worker Roles: Literature Review and Expert Group Survey.* Available from: www.hee.nhs.uk/ sites/default/files/documents/DRad%20support%20workforce%20-%20literature%20 review.pdf

HEE (2021b). *Allied Health Professions' Support Worker Competency, Education, and Career Development Framework. Realising Potential to Deliver Confident, Capable Care for the Future.* https://healtheducationengland.sharepoint.com/Comms/Digital/Shared%20Do cuments/Forms/AllItems.aspx?id=%2FComms%2FDigital%2FShared%20Docume nts%2Fhee%2Enhs%2Euk%20documents%2FWebsite%20files%2FAllied%20health%20 professions%2FAHP%5FFramework%20Final%2Epdf&parent=%2FComms%2FDigi tal%2FShared%20Documents%2Fhee%2Enhs%2Euk%20documents%2FWebsite%20fi les%2FAllied%20health%20professions&p=true

Kessler, I., Heron, P. and Dopson, S. (2015). Professionalization and expertise in care work: The hoarding and discarding of tasks in nursing. *Human Resource Management* 54(5), 737–752.

National Health Executive (2013). Healthcare support workers – registration and regula-tion. *Health Service Focus*, March/April 2013. Available from: www.nationalhealthexecut ive.com/Health-Service-Focus/healthcare-support-workers-registration-and-regulation

Nursing and Midwifery Council (2020a). *Delegation. Caring with Confidence. The Code in Action.* Available from: www.nmc.org.uk/standards/code/code-in-action/delegation/

Nursing and Midwifery Council (2020b). *The Code. Professional Standard for Practice for Nurses, Midwives and Nursing Associates.* Available from: www.nmc.org.uk/globalassets/sitedo cuments/nmc-publications/nmc-code.pdf

Potter, P., Deshields, T. and Marilee, K. (2010). Delegation practices between registered nurses and nursing assistive personnel. *Journal of Nursing Management* 18(2), 157–165. https://doi.org/10.1111/j.1365-2834.2010.01062.x

Pringle, S. A. (2017). The challenges of upskilling health care assistants in community nursing. *British Journal of Community Nursing* 22(6), 284–288. https://doi.org/10.12968/ bjcn.2017.22.6.284

RCM. (2011). *The Role and Responsibilities of MSWs*. RCM. Available at: www.rcm.org.uk/media/2338/role-responsibilities-maternity-support-workers.pdf

RCN (2022). *Accountability and Delegation*. Available from: www.rcn.org.uk/professional-development/accountability-and-delegation

Richards, M. (2020). *Diagnostics: Recovery and Renewal*. Available from: www.england.nhs.uk/wp-content/uploads/2020/10/BM2025Pu-item-5-diagnostics-recovery-and-renewal.pdf

Shore, B., Maben, J., Mold, F., Winkey, K., Cook, A. and Stenner, K. (2020). Delegation of medication administration from registered nurses to non-registered support workers in community care settings: A systematic review with critical interpretive synthesis. *International Journal of Nursing Studies* 126. https://doi.org/10.1016/j.ijnurstu.2021.104121

Snowdon, D. A., Storr, B., Davis, A., Taylor, N. F. and William, C. F. (2020) The effect of delegation of therapy to allied health assistants on patient and organisational outcomes: a systematic review and meta-analysis. *BMC Health Services Research*. DOI: 10.1186/s12913-020-05312-4

Tardivel, J. (2012). Role of the healthcare assistant in an acute setting. *British Journal of Healthcare Assistants* 6(11), 550–555. https://doi.org/10.12968/bjha.2012.6.11.550

PART IV

Go further

7

WIDENING PARTICIPATION INTO HEALTHCARE DEGREES AND DEGREE APPRENTICESHIPS

Introduction

Assessing the rising demand for diagnostic radiography services and the shortage of qualified radiographers, Halliday and colleagues (2020) stated that there 'should be no barriers to staff joining as Band 2 and progressing up to Band 8' (p. 9). In reality, and although many support workers would like to progress into pre-registration degrees work-based routes into registered grades in the NHS are underdeveloped. Barriers do exist. These barriers include a lack of clear information and guidance and sufficient recognition of existing staff's experience and vocational qualifications by universities (Bateson et al., 2016).

This chapter will consider these barriers and what needs to be done so that support workers are able to 'Go Further' and complete the last stage of a GYO workforce approach by moving Inside/Up. Without wishing to confuse you even more by adding yet another label to our lexicon of workforce strategy, a major feature of the Go Further career stage is what is described as 'widening participation'. As so often with workforce strategy this is not a straightforward concept.

What is widening participation?

Widening participation (or sometimes 'widening access') is an important facet of Inside/Up GYO approaches to workforce planning. Reviewing the literature, both Kaehene and colleagues (2014), Bateson and colleagues (2016) and Heaslip and colleagues (2017) noted that there is a lack of agreement in healthcare about what it exactly means with, for example NHS employers interpreting it differently to Higher Education Institutions (HEIs). Support workers (and other targeted groups) tend to be unfamiliar with the term all together (Bateson et al., 2016). This lack of consensus means that there can be a tension between employers, who would

DOI: 10.4324/9781003251620-14

like to see more flexible entry-requirements to help their support staff train to be registered staff, and HEIs, who are 'concerned that candidates will not meet the academic standards demanded' (Bateson et al., 2016: 7).

I define 'widening participation' as an objective (end point) with linked activities that seeks to attract and support under-represented groups into healthcare degrees. Groups may be underrepresented in respect of their gender, disability, socio-economic status, age or ethnicity (Bateson et al., 2016; Heaslip et al., 2017). People who began their NHS career as support workers are underrepresented in registered grades given the proportions who would like to progress (see Table 7.1). Such workers may demonstrate other characteristics of underrepresented groups such as age and socio-economic status (see Chapter 2). A 'catalogue' of interventions exists to support widening participation (The Sutton Trust, 2015: 1). These include ambassadors, day schools and outreach teams. In many ways widening participation mirrors the Outside/InGYO approaches discussed in Chapter 3 – both are concerned with supporting underrepresented groups.

The NHS and widening participation

Much of the recent focus on widening participation in the NHS stems from the decision in 2010 to make nursing an all-graduate profession. Writing at the time, Glasper (2010) argued that this could reduce the diversity of nursing. The 'profession…needs talented and skilled people from all backgrounds and diverse educational achievement to provide the quality-of-care tomorrow's patients will expect' (p. 925). Camilla Cavendish (2013) argued that support workers need a 'simple… career ladder' allowing them to progress into pre-registration degrees – 'not least because support workers would make great nurses, occupational therapists and social workers' (p. 59). Creating work-based routes into healthcare degrees and degree apprenticeships delivers a range of benefits as well as fulfilling the aspirations of those not insignificant numbers of support workers who wish to become registered

TABLE 7.1 The proportion of the support workforce wishing to progress into pre-registration

Occupational group	Proportion (%)	Source
Radiography	45	Snaith et al., 2018
Maternity wishing to become midwives	18.9	Griffin, 2018
Maternity wishing to become nurses	4.7	Griffin, 2018
Mental health	46	Griffin, 2021
Nursing	'A third'	Glasper, 2010
Nursing	17.9–29.6	Kessler et al., 2019
Other professions	4.7–10.1	Kessler et al., 2019
Nursing Associates wishing to become nurses	75	Kessler et al., 2021b
Nursing support workers wishing to become nurses or Nursing Associates	46	Kessler et al., 2021a

staff. These benefits include–reduced vacancies, a more diverse student population and a more stable workforce because students who have previously been support workers are likely to remain working for their host NHS trust, following graduation (Department of Health, 2010).

There is a lack of research on health care widening participation programmes including those focused on existing employees (Kaehene et al., 2014; Smith et al., 2015; Bateson et al., 2016; Heaslip et al., 2017). A consequence of this lack of evidence base, coupled with a lack of data, is that 'efforts to expand pilot models and share good practice' are impeded in the NHS (Bateson et al., 2016: 6).

How many support workers wish to enter pre-registration healthcare degrees?

Drawn from available research, Table 7.1 sets out the proportion of support workers, employed in different occupations, who report that they would like to become registered healthcare professionals. Glasper's (2010) statement that 'a third of HCAs aspire to enter the nursing register' (p. 955) is not referenced, although it is not out of line with Kessler and colleagues (2019) case study assessments of support worker career aspirations. Kessler and colleagues (2021a) more recent survey of nearly 4,000 nursing support workers found that 46% wished to progress into either Nursing Associate or registered nursing roles. Griffin (2018, 2021) and Snaith and colleagues (2018) estimates are based on national surveys of support workers.

Kessler and colleagues (2021) survey of Nursing Associates and Trainee Nursing Associates found that 75% aspired to become registered nurses – a percentage which is striking – but this high figure more than likely reflects the fact that the Nursing Associate role was, at least in part, developed explicitly as a step into nursing degrees (Willis, 2015). Although not explicitly designed for the purpose there is also some evidence that foundation degrees have also been used primarily as a means to progress into pre-registration (Miller et al., 2015). This might explain the high proportion of Assistant Practitioners, Snaith and colleagues (2018) identified as wishing to become radiographers.

The available evidence, although it varies, suggests that a significant minority of the clinical support workforce aspire to become registered professionals. Assuming conservatively that a fifth of the support workforce in the NHS aspire to be registered staff, this represents, nationally, a potential pool of an additional 86,000 staff. By way of comparison in 2021 around 70,000 NHS employees were EU nationals (House of Commons, 2021).

The benefits of widening participation

Mahsood and colleagues (2017) review of the evidence more generally on the impact of widening participation, identified advantages for individuals (in the form of higher wages and increased confidence), employers (improved productivity) and society as a whole (social mobility and cohesion). Turning to the evidence specifically from healthcare, Heaslip and colleagues (2017) reported that NHS employers liked widening participation students, who had gone through the apprenticeship route, because they could 'hit the ground running' (p. 72). In their review of the peer review literature and in a critical review of a series of NHS widening participation programmes, Bateson and colleagues (2016) noted that the motivation of the organisations engaged in widening participation was a moral one – a 'belief' in the importance of widening participation for underrepresented groups (p. 6). Reviewing the evidence for widening participation into nurse education, Heaslip and colleagues (2017) identified benefits deriving from widening participation for the delivery of learning. It 'enriches the learning', they wrote, through 'promoting values such as equality and tolerance and diversifying the social and cultural environment', (p. 67). They conclude that 'widening participation is not only important for patient care; it is a fundamental mechanism to address workforce issues' (p. 68).

BOX 7.1 WIDENING PARTICIPATION INTO NURSING

In response to nursing becoming an all-graduate profession in 2010, the Department of Health published guidance on how existing NHS support staff might be supported into pre-registration degrees. Camilla Cavendish (2013) replicated the models in her review. The rationale for work-based widening participation, the Department of Health (2010) stated were:

- To build capacity to meet rising demand for services.
- Ensuring that a diverse workforce was recruited into nursing.
- Ensuring the nursing workforce reflected the communities it served.
- Supporting a stable workforce.

Glasper (2010) noted that 'critics of the ... decision to develop an all-graduate nursing workforce have complained that the new changes will restrict entry to the profession and put academic study above practical work, caring and compassion' (p. 924).

Unison (2008) found some evidence that widening participation students had lower attrition rates on nursing degrees than more traditional students, Heaslip and colleagues' (2017) literature review however found just one other study investigating attrition and widening participation on healthcare degrees. This suggested that students who enter HEIs via an access course (see below) may in fact have a higher quit rate than A Level or BTEC students, although this was not statistically significant. They also note that individuals studying access courses a more likely to be mature and/or from a BAME group which might explain quit rates rather than the access course itself. A recent study focused on the student population as a whole found that BTEC students were twice as likely to drop out of a degree programme before their second year than A Level students (Dilnot and Macmillan, 2022). This finding perhaps underlines the importance of continuing support once underrepresented groups start studying on degree courses (Bateson et al., 2016). The report (op. cit.) also highlights that BTECs are an effective route into higher education for students from lower socio-economic backgrounds.

The case for why degree students drawn from the NHS clinical support workforce *should* have higher completion and retention rates on graduating can be made. Support workers have occupationally relevant knowledge, skills and attitudes, along with experience of the physical and emotional demands of working in healthcare. On graduating they are likely to remain working for their host NHS trust. They are also familiar with the way the NHS operates, such as weekend working and long shifts, and the demands of care. There is evidence, for example, that one of the factors contributing to students leaving radiography degrees and for the high turnover in the early days of employment is 'compassion fatigue' (Flinton et al., 2018). The emotional pressures arising from working in radiography can be a particular issue for young people who have not yet developed coping mechanisms to deal with the demands of the profession (ibid.). It is striking that around half of radiography Assistant Practitioners, wish to become registered radiographers (Snaith et al., 2018). It is not unreasonable to consider that that experience and knowledge, as HEE (2021) suggest that they possess should mean that radiography support staff, would be more likely to be able to cope with the emotional demands of radiography. For nursing, we have already discussed in Chapter 3, the 'transition shock' that newly qualified staff can feel when first becoming registered practitioners.

BOX 7.2 ACCESS COURSES AND HIGHER NATIONALS

Many FE providers deliver *Access to Higher Education Diploma* courses. These RQF level 3 qualifications aim to provide students with sufficient credits and knowledge to apply for university courses, perhaps because they do not have a traditional qualification like an A Level. Any course containing 'Access to Higher Education' in its title must be recognised by the Quality Assurance Agency for Higher Education. In 2017–2018 some 37,000 students completed Access Courses, with 20,000 of these subsequently accessed university courses (The Quality Assurance Agency for Higher Education, 2021).

There are many courses available aimed at aspiring healthcare students, such as *Access to HE Diploma in Nursing and Midwifery, Access to HE Diploma Allied Health Professions* or *Access to Radiography*. Typically, these courses teach general study skills, such as research or digital skills, along with general healthcare subjects such as human biology and the physiological aspects of health and occupationally specific knowledge such as, for radiography, cell structure and function.

Higher Nationals are qualifications at RQF levels 4 and 5 – the equivalent to the first and second year of a degree course. Higher Nationals have been co-designed with industry, HEIs and FE providers. As with Access Courses, there are Higher Nationals specifically for those wishing to pursue a career in healthcare.

Barriers to widening participation

In their review of the research, Bateson and colleagues (2016) identified the following barriers that NHS support workers who aspire to train to be a registered professional might face:

- A lack of clear of information and guidance.
- Lack of support from managers.
- Affordability, particularly because support worker candidates are more likely to be mature employees with financial commitments such as mortgages.
- Concerns about managing study and other commitments such as caring responsibilities.
- Lack of functional skills.
- A lack of parity between A levels and equivalent vocational qualifications.
- The complexity of navigating HEI entrance procedures without support and which vary between institutions.
- Lack of clear work-based progression routes.

There is evidence that admission tutors, (and indeed other university students), view vocational qualifications such as BTECs, as being inferior to A levels even though they are equivalent (Shields and Masardo, 2015). Degrees do though require rigorous study and HEIs rightly expect potential students to possess sufficient qualifications to meet the demands of a healthcare courses. Interestingly though the same emphasis does not appear to be placed on the potential of students to cope with the placement element of degrees, one of the main reasons why students leave (see Griffin, 2019).

There is limited evidence of support worker's experience of academic study. However, a survey of over 500 Nursing Associates, discussed in more detail below, found that the nature of study (an apprenticeship centred on a completing a RQF level 5 foundation degree delivered by a HEI), for most trainees was an 'intense and perhaps difficult process' (Kessler et al., 2021: 19). One of the elements of the apprenticeship trainees found most demanding was completing academic assignments, although the most demanding, cited by 53% of the sample, was finding time to study. The two findings may be linked.

Support workers seeking to progress their careers also face structural barriers. As we saw in Chapter 5 apprenticeships are increasingly becoming the main way that NHS support workers access formal learning. There are numerous apprenticeships at RQF level 3 that are relevant to NHS clinical and non-clinical support workers ranging from apprenticeship standards in *Advanced Carpentry and Joinery* to *Workplace Pensions Consultant* and *Administrator.* Many are designed to upskill clinical support staff, not least the *Senior Healthcare Support Worker* standard, which covers nursing, theatre staff, maternity support workers and therapy support staff. HEI degree courses require a minimum of a RQF level 3 qualification, which these apprenticeships provide, along with the necessary level of functional skills, elements of study skills and occupationally relevant learning. However, the qualification element of the apprenticeships is set at 60 credits. For many HEIs, 60 credits are not sufficient to enter their degree programmes. The gap between RQF level 3 apprenticeship credits and UCAS points has been a long-standing issue in the NHS (Turnbin et al., 2019). If HEIs are not willing to take account of experiential learning (see below), then support workers will either need to complete a RQF level 4 or 5 apprenticeship, such as the Assistant Practitioner one which does have sufficient credits or find another way to bridge the gap.

Which widening participation interventions work?

There are a substantial number of interventions designed to widen participation into Higher Education (The Sutton Trust, 2015). These include: access courses, study skill programmes, summer schools, mentors, role models, ambassadors, campus visits and outreach teams. There is, though, 'very little evidence which…initiatives are most effective' (ibid., 1). There is some evidence that early exposure to nursing, for example through work experience, has a positive impact on applications for a nursing degree (Smith et al., 2016). This study focused on young people, however, not existing support staff reflecting a wider absence of widening participation research aimed at existing employees (Bateson et al., 2016).

The Sutton Trust (2015) reviewed the evidence for the efficacy of the various interventions. Although not from the perspective of healthcare, it is likely that interventions that successfully widen participation for non-healthcare degrees would be effective for healthcare too. It should be noted that these strategies can also assist with recruitment more widely as part of the Outside/In GYO approaches discussed in Chapter 3. The interventions identified as being effective were:

- The provision of information and support in respect of applications.
- Financial support.
- Mentoring.
- Open days.
- Residential schemes.
- Support to meet attainment levels.

There is some evidence from the NHS for the positive benefits of open days, mentors and extended support on employment for new support worker recruits (Cavendish, 2013). Bateson and colleagues (2016) identified factors characterising an effective approach to widening participation in the NHS, based on interviews with NHS trusts and HEIs operating widening participation programmes:

- Collaboration and partnership between employers and education providers.
- Key individuals in NHS trusts are engaged and committed to widening participation.
- Support interventions are consistent, well-planned, and sustained.
- Engagement with target groups is on-going.
- Widening participation extends from application to retention, completion, and employment. It is a process not an event.

Why have widening participation interventions not been mobilised extensively in the NHS?

Given the long-standing shortages of registered staff in the NHS, and the recommendations of both the Cavendish (2013) and Willis (2015) reviews, along with HEE's *Talent for Care* (2014a) and *Widening Participation* strategies (2014b), it is perhaps surprising that support staff still face significant barriers when seeking to access pre-registration degrees. No systematic research has been undertaken as to why this might be, although Turbin and colleagues (2019) asserted that this may be due to a policy focus 'that stresses efficiencies – efficiency means skill mix' (p. 172) rather than career progression, although as we have seen (see Linay and Lloyd, 2020) for example), there is no evidence that registered roles have been replaced by support worker ones. Indeed, the government continues to stress the importance of recruiting registered staff as the 2020 pledge to recruit 50,000 additional nurses (Ford, 2020) illustrates. The most likely reason why barriers still exist is, once again, a lack of a systematic approach to the problems. HEIs can set their own entry-requirements and decide whether to recognise experiential learning or not. Funding is not available to assist support workers who wish to progress. This problem was particularly recognised by Lord Willis (2015) in his review of nurse education, and his proposal for addressing it – the creation of a new bridging support role called the Nursing Associate.

Nursing Associates

The Nursing Associate role was introduced into the NHS in 2017, following the recommendation in the Willis (2015) review. The role was designed specifically to create a bridge between support roles in nursing and nursing degrees, although the role can also act as a senior support worker role in its own right. Nursing Associates work in all the branches of nursing (adult, children, mental health and learning disabilities) and in all settings (acute, community, mental health, general practice and social care). Normally graded at *Agenda for Change* band 4 (and band 3 during their training, which last two years). Nursing Associates can perform a wide range of tasks, following training, including:

- The administration of intravenous drugs.
- Wound care.
- Venepuncture.
- ECGs.
- Supporting individuals and their families through unwelcome news.
- Clinical observations and measurements such as pulse and temperature.

Nursing Associates complete the RQF level 5 apprenticeship linked to the role, which contains a foundation degree. On completion Nursing Associates, are then able to complete the Nursing Degree Apprenticeship (see below) in two years, recognising that the foundation degree's curriculum covers the same content as the early part of a nursing degree.

As with all apprenticeships Nursing Associates combine 'off-the-job' study with work-based learning and are assessed through an integrated End Point Assessment process. Nursing Associates are required to complete a minimum of 460 hours of external practice placement. The title, 'Nursing Associate' is protected, and the role regulated by the Nursing and Midwifery Council. Trainees rotate across several placement areas, but retain a base area that they spend most of their work-based learning time in.

In 2021 there were 4,000 registered Nursing Associates employed in the NHS and a further 6,000 trainees (Kessler et al., 2021a). A survey of nursing support workers found that 14% had or were undertaking the Nursing Associate apprenticeship or an Assistant Practitioner one (ibid.). A further 40% of the sample indicated that they would be interested in training to be a Nursing Associate or commencing the Nurse Degree apprenticeship (Kessler and colleagues, 2021b, 2022). Kessler and colleagues (2021a) note that there 'continues to be much debate on the nature and consequences of the Nursing Associate role, which in the absence of strong evidence has often been impressionistic, anecdotal and in some cases speculative' (p. 4).

Kessler and his colleagues at King's College London (2021a) surveyed 516 Nursing Associates and trainee Nursing Associates to gain their views on the role, their training and deployment (see Chapter 1 for the survey's findings on the demographic characteristics of the Nursing Associate workforce). It found a mixed picture. Despite expectations that trainees would be supernumerary, 12% of those responding to the survey said they were not when outside of their base placement, and 74% said that they were not supernumerary on their base placement. Perhaps not surprisingly, given the dual purpose of the role as a bridge into pre-registration and a stand-alone support role, Nursing Associates are 'only gradually finding a place in established care delivery routines and becoming understood and appreciated by colleagues' (Kessler et al., 2021a: 24). Drawing on the Institutional Model of New Roles we discussed in Chapter 2, Nursing Associates might be said to be at the 'Legitimacy' stage where, for example, their value needs to be proven to others (Kessler et al., 2017). A sign of this is that, despite the role being framed by the Nursing and Midwifery Council *Standards of Proficiency*, its scope of practice Kessler and colleagues found (ibid.) is still 'very much "work-in-practice"' (p. 34). This is not just true for those working with the Nursing Associates, but for the Nursing Associates themselves. Over one in ten (13%) of qualified Nursing Associates said that they did not understand the role 'at all', and 41% that they only partly understood it. Kessler and colleagues (ibid.) quote Nursing Associates who told them, 'I feel my role is extremely new within my service and they don't know how best to utilise my skills and knowledge' and '[m]ost managers do not know what is allowed within my role' (p. 24).

These quotes reflect a further finding which was that the tasks Nursing Associates performed varied considerably. For example, just 4% administered intravenous drugs and 13% carried out a first visit to someone's house. In contrast, 66% made beds and 76% carried out observations. Despite being nationally designed with a single qualification, the Nursing Associate role, like other support workers still lacked consistency and standardisation and was poorly understood and unevenly valued. Deployment of the role is not yet consistent with the key tasks that distinguish it from Assistant Practitioners – particularly drug administration – being performed in only a minority of cases (Kessler et al., 2021b). The value of the role may, then, be more as a step into nursing, as *Shape of Caring* (Willis, 2015) intended than as an enhanced support worker role.

How to widen access into pre-registration programmes

We have seen that a significant minority of support workers would like to progress into registered grades and that there are potential benefits in assisting them to do so. These staff represent a largely untapped future supply of registered staff. In this section we will discuss how workplace routes can be mobilised to enable widening participation, including the role of Degree Apprenticeships.

It is worth considering again Bateson and colleagues (2016) finding that a key characteristic of successful widening participation is partnership and collaboration. ICSs create an ideal opportunity to bring all partners – employers, FE, ITPs and HEIs – together to develop a progression agreement. Traditionally progression agreements have focused on enabling learners on FE delivered vocational courses access specific HEI courses. An example of this would be colleges that deliver the Health Technical Level agreeing with a local HEI that students who completed the T Level could be guaranteed an interview for a healthcare degree. The agreements can also acknowledge that people with specific higher-level qualifications, like foundation degrees, do not need to repeat that study when they join a degree course. Progression agreements can also include employers, and recognition of work-based programmes like RQF level 3 apprenticeships as well as agreeing any mechanisms necessary to support employees to apply for courses.

Work-base progression routes into healthcare degrees

There are a number of paths that *could* be pursued by existing support workers into healthcare degrees. Figure 7.1 is an updated and adapted from the 2010 Department

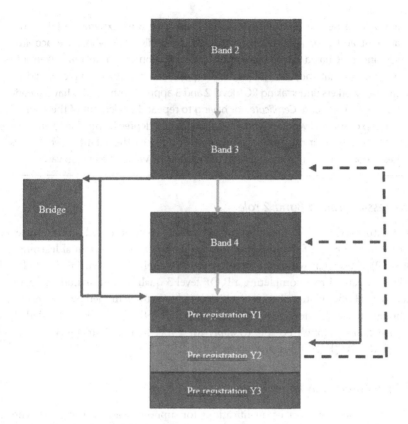

FIGURE 7.1 Progression routes.

of Health widening participation models and Cavendish's (2013) model both of which I developed. It is founded on *Agenda for Change* bands and assumes staff at band 2 possess RQF level 2 qualifications, band 3, RQF level 3 and band 4, RQF level 4 or 5, although this may not always be the case.

BOX 7.3 ACCREDITATION AND RECOGNITION OF PRIOR AND EXPERIENTIAL LEARNING

Accreditation and Recognition of Prior and Experiential Learning (APEL) or Recognition of Prior Learning (RPL) refers to the potential of education providers to consider formal learning that does not result in a qualification. An example would be *The Care Certificate* or in-work training courses, as well as informal learning acquired through work or personal experience. The life experience of someone who has been a carer, could be taken into account.

APEL enables widening participation in two ways. Firstly, it can mean that support workers (and others) who may not possess necessary qualifications to apply for a degree (or sufficient credits) can have their experience taken into account and their application considered. Secondly, staff who have acquired learning that has a direct bearing on a qualification can have that taken into account so that they do not have to repeat learning. An example would be support workers undertaking RQF level 2 and 3 apprenticeships who have already undertaken *The Care Certificate* not having to repeat that element of the apprenticeship or support workers who have a foundation degree being able to advance to the second year of a healthcare degree (or further). The extent to which HEIs take prior learning into account and the process by which they do so varies.

Progression from a Band 2 role

Staff with a RQF level 2 qualification are unlikely to be accepted on to a university course on the basis of that qualification alone even with experiential learning (see Box 7.3). These staff will need to either progress their career within the NHS initially to a band 3 role completing a RQF level 3 qualification or study an external Access or Higher National course, which is unlikely to be funded by their employer although I have come across examples of where NHS trusts have funded these. Such staff may though be able to apply for a role such as Nursing Associate and complete a RQF level 5 qualification.

Progression from a Band 3 role

The key issue in respect of qualifications for support workers in band 3 who do not possess three A levels is whether the university they are interested in applying to recognises the qualifications they might possess, such as NVQs or BTECs. As we have already discussed the credits associated with the *Senior Healthcare Support Worker* apprenticeship may fall short in terms of UCAS tariff entry-requirements. In some areas the content of the apprenticeship may also be seen as insufficient, compared to students with for example science A levels. HEIs do have the option to take account of experience and experiential learning (Box 7.3), but they do not have too. Like band 2 support workers, staff in this position could study on an external access course or if the opportunity arose progress to band 4 role. There are also a limited number of bridging programmes available (see box below).

Band 3 staff that do have sufficient qualifications and/or whose experience is recognised could join either a traditional undergraduate degree or the degree apprenticeship, if one is available for their chosen profession in the same way that A Level students do.

Progression from Band 4s

Band 4 staff who possess a RQF level 4 or 5 qualification will have sufficient UCAS points to apply to the first year of their chosen degree. Those with a level

5 qualification such as a foundation degree should be able to APEL into the at least the second year of the degree in most subjects (maternity is an exception, Griffin, 2018).

Progression into support roles

Many healthcare degree courses experience high attrition rates with, for example one in four nursing students dropping out of their course before they graduate (Health Foundation, 2018) for a range of reasons including cost of living (Collins, 2019). This obviously represents a considerable loss of potential staff for the NHS. The progression model allows for such students to step off of their degree course and work, instead, as a healthcare support worker.

BOX 7.4 NHS BRIDGING PROGRAMMES

Bridging programmes, like access courses, provide formal accredited learning that allows people whose qualifications do not either provide sufficient credits or cover the subjects required for a degree, or both, to meet that gap. In 2015 Skills for Health developed a specific programme for healthcare workers the aim of which was to, in 'combination with a relevant level 3 vocational qualification', provide 'another route for people in the healthcare support workforce who wish to progress into nursing and other health professional educational programmes at universities in England' (Skills for Health, 2015: 3) Successful completion of the Bridging Programme leads to the *RQF Level 3 Certificate in Bridging Skills for Higher Education.* The programme was not funded, and take-up appears to have been minimal probably for this reason. The programme is no longer featured on the Skills for Health website but is the RQF level 3 qualification is available for delivery.

Degree apprenticeships

Healthcare degree apprenticeships were introduced in 2017. They are structured in exactly the same way as other apprenticeships combining work and study (see Chapter 5) and funded through the apprenticeship levy. They are an opportunity to obtain a bachelor's degree (RQF level 6) or masters (RQF level 7) through a work-based route. Given that the average student debt totalled in 2020 totalled £45,000 (House of Commons Library, 2019b) degree apprenticeships are an attractive option, including for support workers who, as we have seen, are likely to have existing financial commitments.

The degree that apprentices gain is exactly the same as that traditional under-graduate students' study, covering the same curriculum and meeting the requirements of registration with regulatory bodies such as the Nursing and Midwifery Council.

The 'off-the-job' study can be through day or block release, be in person or virtual and is protected through supernumerary status. As with other apprenticeships the levy cannot be used to cover backfill costs, although employers benefit from the apprentices working for them as support workers during their study. The rate at which apprentices are paid is left to the discretion of local employers (the minimum legally that can be paid is the National Minimum Wage). A wide range of approaches have been adopted by employers – spot pay, the National Minimum Wage, the apprentice's previous salary if already employed in the NHS or Annex 21 of *Agenda for Change* paying a set proportion of the substantive grades' pay (Alma Economics, 2020). Degree apprenticeships typically last four years but can be three years long.

Blended Learning Degrees

Introduced in 2020 for nursing and 2021 for midwifery, Blended Learning Degrees (BLDs) maximise the use of digital technologies. Using Augmented Reality, Virtual Reality, simulation, gaming, and virtual learning environments the vast majority of academic learning (up to 95%) takes place online, with students only occasionally accessing campuses at their chosen university. Even a proportion of the student's placements can be virtual through the use of simulation. HEE hoped that BLDs will not only support a growth in the nursing or midwifery workforce but also widen participation and create a more digitally expert workforce, recognising the growing use of digital technology in healthcare.

BOX 7.5 FLIPPED CLASSROOMS

BLDs are an example of a 'flipped classroom'. Traditionally students would attend lectures to be taught about a subject. Flipped classrooms turn this traditional approach on its head with students first encountering the material through virtual learning environments and later attending classes (which could be virtual as well) to enhance their understanding.

Conclusion

Many support workers would like to progress their careers into registered grades but often face barriers to doing so, such as a lack of recognition of their work experience or a paucity of information and support to assist their application. This means that the NHS misses the opportunity to take advantage of GYO routes into the professions which would bring a number of benefits to services and the NHS. It is possible to chart progression work-based routes into pre-registration degrees and apprenticeships provide pathways for most occupations. Degree apprenticeships and other new ways of studying a degree enable support staff with caring, financial, and other responsibilities to access HE. ICS-wide progression agreements create the opportunity for HEIs, FE providers, employers and others to explicitly recognise the importance of GYO and support NHS employees, as well as externally underrepresented groups, into healthcare degrees.

Checklist

* Is information available to support workers about the work-based pathways they could follow into pre-registration healthcare degrees?
* Are support workers who are able to apply for healthcare degrees supported to do so?
* Are employers clear about the purpose of Nursing Associates? Is the role a senior support staff one or a step into nursing or both? Does workforce planning reflect this?
* Do local HEIs acknowledge and support work based routes into pre-registration, particularly from *Agenda for Change* band 3 roles? If not, why not and what needs to be done to support access?
* At ICS level do all education providers (HEIs, colleges and ITPs) work together with employers and the ICS to widen access into pre-registration?
* Is there a progression agreement?

References

Alma Economics (2019). *Apprenticeships.* HEE (unpublished).

Bateson, J., Griffin, R., Somerville, M., Hancock, D. and Proctor, S. (2016). *Different People, Different Views, Different Ideas: Widening Participation in Nursing and Radiography Degrees.* Institution of Vocational Learning and Workforce Learning, Bucks New University.

Cavendish, C. (2013). *Cavendish Review. An Independent Enquiry into Healthcare Assistants and Support Workers in the NHS and Social Care Settings.* London, Department of Health. Available from: https://assets.publishing.service.gov.uk/government/uploads/system/uploads/attachment_data/file/236212/Cavendish_Review.pdf

Collins, A. (2019). 'Cost of living' main reason student nurses drop out. *Health Service Journal,* 11 November 2019. Available from: www.hsj.co.uk/workforce/cost-of-living-main-reason-why-student-nurses-drop-out/7026285.article?mkt_tok=eyJpIjoiWVdkKaFpUa3dPRFExT0dNMyIsInQiOiJwWVVHRzVuNkpcL0VKRmdCSkQ0Ung0R1wvWHRVdktQTXVQZkN0RldtcmdkOVwvK2NmMGhTNkNHb3hFWjZTG1la2NaKzBlYY0lwQU9UdEQ2UjViYUppVG8zOUJYcStvWm1DaXdaaVEtcL0dpRm52OVRKRGR2Q3BZblF6NXdkVVBDSENENxOXkifQ%3D%3D

Department of Health (2010). *Widening Participation in Pre-registration Nursing Programmes.* Available from: https://assets.publishing.service.gov.uk/government/uploads/system/uploads/attachment_data/file/213867/dh_116655.pdf

Dilnot, C. and Macmillan, L. (2022). *Educational Choices at 16-19 and Adverse Outcomes at University.* Nuffield Foundation. Available from: www.nuffieldfoundation.org/project/educational-choices-at-16-19-and-adverse-outcomes-at-university

Flinton, D., Cherry, P., Thorne, R., Mannion, L., O'Sullivan, C. and Khine, R. (2018). Compassion satisfaction and fatigue: an investigation into levels being reported by radiotherapy students. *Journal of Radiotherapy in Practice* 17, 364–367.

Ford, M. (2020). Government's 50,000 more nurses target 'insufficient for growing demand'. *Nursing Times*. www.nursingtimes.net/news/workforce/governments-50000-more-nur ses-target-insufficient-for-growing-demand-09-12-2020/

Glasper, A. (2010) Widening participation in pre-registration nursing. *British Journal of Nursing* 19(4), 924–925.

Griffin, R. (2018). *The Deployment, Education and Development of Maternity Support Workers in England. A Scoping Report to Health Education England. RCM*. Available from: www.rcm. org.uk/media/2347/the-deployment-education-and-development-of-maternity-supp ort-workers-in-england.pdf

Griffin, R. (2020). *Partnerships and Pathways. Creating New Supply Routes to Build Capacity and Capability in Therapeutic Radiography. A Report to HEE*. Unpublished. London, King's College London.

Griffin, R. (2021). *A Rewarding Job, but Frustrating Career. The Education, Development, and Deployment of Clinical Support Workers Employed in NHS Mental Health Services*. King's College London

Halliday, K., Maskell, G., Beeley, L. and Quick, E. (2020). *Radiology. GIRFT Programme National Speciality Report*. Available from: www.gettingitrightfirsttime.co.uk/wp-cont ent/uploads/2020/11/GIRFT-radiology-report.pdf

Health Foundation (2018). *One in Four Student Nurses Drop Out of Their Degrees before Graduation*. Available from: www.health.org.uk/news-and-comment/news/one-in-four-student-nurses-drop-out-of-their-degrees-before-graduation

Heaslip, V., Board, M., Duckworth, V. and Thomas, L. (2017). Widening participation in nurse education: An integrative literature. *Nurse Education Today* 59, 66–74. DOI: 10.1016/ j.nedt.2017.08.016.Epub 2017 Sep 14.

HEE (2014a). *Talent for Care. A National Strategic Framework to Develop the Healthcare Support Workforce*. Available from: www.hee.nhs.uk/sites/default/files/documents/TfC%20Natio nal%20Strategic%20Framework_0.pdf

HEE (2014b). *Widening Participation It Matters. Our Strategy and Initial Action Plan*. Available from: www.hee.nhs.uk/sites/default/files/documents/Widening%20Participation%20 it%20Matters_0.pdf

House of Commons Library (2021a). *NHS Staffing from Overseas: Statistics*. Available from: https://commonslibrary.parliament.uk/research-briefings/cbp-7783/

House of Commons Library (2021b). *Student Loan Statistics*. Available from: https://com monslibrary.parliament.uk/research-briefings/sn01079/

Kaehne, A., Maden, M., Roe, B., Thomas, L. and Brown, J. (2014). *Literature Review on Approaches and Impact of Interventions to Facilitate Widening Participation in Healthcare Programmes. Health Education North West*. Available from: https://repository.edgehill.ac.uk/ 6200/1/WPlitrev280514Submitted.pdf

Kessler, I., Heron, P. and Spilsbury, K. (2017). Human resource management innovation in health care: the institutionalisation of new support roles. *Human Resource Management Survey* 27(2), 228–245.

Kessler, I., Steils, N., Harris, J. Manthorpe, J. and Moriarty, J. (2021a). *The Development of the Nursing Associate Role: The Postholder Perspective*. NIHR Policy Research Unit in Health and Social Care Workforce The Policy Institute, King's College London.

Kessler, I., Steils, N., Esser, A. and Grant, D. (2021b). Understanding career development and progression from a healthcare support worker perspective Part 1. *British Journal of Healthcare Assistants* 15(11), 526–531. https://doi.org/10.12968/bjha.2021.15.11.526

Kessler, I., Steils, N., Esser, A. and Grant, D. (2022). Understanding career development and progression from a healthcare support worker perspective Part 2. *British Journal of Healthcare Assistants* 16(1), 6–10. https://doi.org/10.12968/bjha.2022.16.1.6

Mahsood, S. and Whiteford, G. (2017). *Bridges, Pathways and Transitions: International Innovations in Widening Participation*. Chandos Publishing. https://doi.org/10.1016/C2016-0-00812-4

Miller, L., Williams, J., Marvell, R. and Tassinari, A. (2015). *Assistant Practitioners in the NHS in England*. Skills for Health. Available from: www.skillsforhealth.org.uk/images/resource-section/reports/Assistant%20Practitioners%20 in%20England%20Report%202015.pdf

The Quality Assurance Agency for Higher Education (2022). *Access to Higher Education*. Available from: www.accesstohe.ac.uk/en/home#

Shields, R. and Masardo, A. (2015). Changing patterns in vocational entry qualifications, student support and outcomes in undergraduate degree programmes. *Higher Education Academy*. Available from: www.heacademy.ac.uk/sites/default/files/resources/Changing%20Patterns%20in%20Vocational%20Entry%20Qualifications.pdf accessed 1/7/2016

Skills for Health (2015). *Executive Summary. Crossing the Bridge: Progress Report on the Skills for Health Bridging Programme*. Available from: www.skillsforhealth.org.uk/images/standards/bridging/SFH%20Bridging%20Programme-ExecSummary-Report%20June%202015.pdf

Smith, A., Beattie, M. and Kyle, R. G. (2015). 'I know exactly what I am going into': recommendations for pre- nursing experience from an evaluation of pre-nursing scholarship in rural Scotland. *Nursing Open* 2(3), 105–118.

Snaith, B., Harris, M. A. and Palmer, D. (2018). A UK Survey exploring the assistant practitioner role across diagnostic imaging: current practice, relationships and challenges to progression. *British Journal of Radiology* 91 (1091). Available from: www.ncbi.nlm.nih.gov/pmc/articles/PMC6475955/

The Sutton Trust (2015). *Evaluating Access*. Available from: www.suttontrust.com/wp-content/uploads/2015/12/Evaluating-Access-Review-Full-Report. pdf

Turbin, J., Fuller, A. and Wintrup, J. (2014). Apprenticeship and progression in the healthcare sector: can labour market theory illuminate barriers and opportunities in contrasting occupations? *Journal of Vocational Education and Training* 66(2), 156–174.

Willis, P. (2015). *Raising the Bar: Shape of Caring, A Review of the Future Education and Training of Registered Nurses and Care Assistants*. Available from: www.hee.nhs.uk/sites/default/files/documents/2348-Shape-of-caring-review-FINAL.pdf

8

WHAT NEXT FOR NHS SUPPORT WORKERS?

Introduction

The year this book was published marked almost a decade after the Cavendish Review (2013) reported. Back then, I would have been surprised and somewhat disappointed to find out ten years later that so many of the problems she identified were still so prevalent. I would though have been pleased to see the development of national competency frameworks and the efforts made in a number of professions to define the role and responsibilities of support workers, as well as the growing number of apprenticeships relevant to this workforce. What next though? What does the future look like for the NHS clinical workforce? Will it be more of the same or will the positive developments be scaled and sustained? In short will the next decade been a repeat of the last or will there be a step change?

In order to gather insights on the future of support workers I sent a survey to a purposively selected sample of individuals who have been or are currently engaged with support worker development, including support workers themselves. Although it is, of course, impossible to predict the future, particularly one where over the next decade there will be at least two new governments, the respondent's understanding and experience of support workers provides rich information (Palinkas et al., 2015). Respondents worked for arm's length bodies, trade unions, professional bodies, in NHS trusts, education providers and the voluntary sector.

Reimaging the NHS clinical support workforce?

Respondents were asked whether they agreed or not that a series of long-standing issues and barriers faced by support workers would improve by 2031. Table 8.1 sets out the responses.

DOI: 10.4324/9781003251620-15

TABLE 8.1 Support worker development in 2031

Issues	Agree (%)	Not Sure (%)	Disagree (%)
Roles and responsibilities will be clearer	74	6	19
There will be clear progression pathways	71	10	6
Support workers will be valued more by the NHS	55	35	10
There will be sufficient funding for their education	32	26	42
Workforce planning will be based on 'one workforce'	26	45	29
Colleges will play a larger role *recruiting* support staff	55	35	10
Colleges will play a larger role *training* support staff	68	29	3
Progression into pre-registration degrees will be easier	58	35	7
There will be more blended learning	77	19	3
Learning will be transferable	84	13	3
Changes in technology will mean the NHS needs fewer support workers	3	19	77
Support workers will possess formal occupationally relevant qualifications	42	45	13
Apprenticeships will be the main way support workers are trained	64	29	6

As can be seen, respondents felt positively that many of the issues that support workers have faced, such as scope of practice, career pathways, progression into pre-registration degrees, and transferable learning will be resolved by 2031. Respondents were less confident that the NHS would see its clinical workforce as a single whole, when undertaking workforce planning or that there would be sufficient funding available for support worker learning needs, perhaps reflected in the fact that less than half thought that support workers would possess formal occupationally relevant qualifications. Most thought apprenticeships would continue to be the main way support workers were educated, with a greater emphasis on blended learning and with colleges playing a bigger role than they do now not only with training but also for recruitment. Slightly over half felt that the NHS would value support workers more in the future than they do now.

There was a clear view that the support workforce would grow in number and that technological developments such as AI would not reduce demand for support workers.

Participants did point out in their response to an open text question that the improvements they expected, and hoped to see, did depend on a number of enablers. 'A lot will depend on whether they have sufficient tenacity and organisational longevity to make policy and get it embedded', one said referring to the role of national policy makers. Another said that improvements will 'only [be] realised with appropriate government support funding'. 'However, while progress is positive the narrative and rhetoric must be accompanied by recurring policy will and associated resource', another pointed out. 'I'd like to see the support workforce reimagined in the way indicated in this survey, but I don't believe that culture will change significantly enough for this to happen. Hierarchy and custom will hinder progression in a similar way to nursing, which is still heavily overshadowed by the medical model.' Much, then depended, on the political will to develop and resource strategies relevant to support workers.

Hybrid roles

There was a consensus that the future would see a move away from profession-specific support roles towards multi-professional ones, whose job requirements are based on patient pathways. Furthermore, there was an expectation, arising from the need for a greater integration between health and social care, that there would be more multi-agency based support roles with hybrid learning to support the development of these roles. The HEE AHP (2021) support worker competency framework, discussed in Chapter 5, is designed to be applicable to blended roles as well as profession specific ones.

Reason for barriers

As well as looking ahead the survey also explored people's perceptions of why barriers to support worker development exist (only 3% of the sample did not think there were problems). Top of the list were – lack of funding (cited by 87% of the sample), lack of management capacity (77%), poor workforce planning (71%), a lack of valuing of this workforce (61%) and poor-quality appraisals (58%). Regarded as less important were concerns registered staff might have that support staff would replace them (45% thought this was a problem), that support worker learning and development was too complicated (42%), that employers had too much discretion (35%) or that there was a concern about patient safety (26%), all issues that were more significant in the past.

In a free text question, a number of respondents raised the issue of the esteem that support workers are held in locally as being a significant issue:

> 'It links to culture, but I believe support workers are seen undertaking menial tasks and that investing in their development is seen as a waste of resources. In reality they're the eyes and ears of the care system and need the most investment as they spend more time delivering care than many others.'

> 'Support Workers are often viewed as disposable and easily replaceable. The training new recruits receive is often the minimum employers can get away with done as quickly and cheaply as possible.'

'…support workers should not be seen as an afterthought when considering workforce planning and transformation activities.

'They are not appropriately acknowledged as an individual in their own workplace most times and desires of further development is often dismissed by colleagues. Though they are performing tasks and duties such as hygienic support and nutritional support, for example, for service recipients, these duties are dismissed as average and "have to do" without the notion of importance and often there is a lack of understanding why this task has to be done and explained that it's part of the job.'

One respondent also highlighted that the NHS workforce is not treated as one, compounded again by a lack of understanding of what support staff do.

There are very limited/parallel processes employed for the development of support staff which means that the read across to registered or regulated occupations is not always well understood; there is very little acknowledgement of the benefits of a support workforce across the whole of health and care.

What else needs to change?

Respondents to the survey identified a number of other improvements and developments that they would like to see:

- The creation of more senior support worker roles. 'With the increase in confidence of the system re delegation/supervision, and increased capability/capacity of the support workforce, there will be the emergence of more senior support worker roles operating within clinical pathways, taking on more complex roles within the parameters of that clinical pathway and working as part of the [Multi Disciplinary Team].'
- Updating of *Agenda for Change* Job Profiles.
- Formal regulation of all support workers.
- Completion of *The Care Certificate* to be mandatory.
- Greater use of competency frameworks to ensure consistency in job design and deployment. 'Roles and responsibilities of the support workforce vary too much between trusts–much more defined frameworks around these aspects would help with this and would ultimately assist with increasing national parity in the efficient use of support workers overall.'

Respondents were able to articulate a vision of what 'good' would look like for support worker development. One support worker said:

we should have clear knowledge and skills passports, roles and responsibilities, delegation policies, governance structures and discretion re school grade expectations/entry level barriers to progression (many fear they lack academic prowess! but are exceptional vocational workers), we need more compassion in how we support the support workforce.

Another said that there was a need for a

more transparent, efficient and equitable process for the development of support workers is required so retention can be improved and support workers can feel the value of their contribution to quality patient care. Recruitment strategies need to include widening participation principles so we can develop a workforce that meets the needs and in some ways reflects the population they serve.

One workforce

For much of its history the NHS has struggled to ensure it has enough staff with the right skills working in the right place – the core objective of workforce planning. Mostly the NHS has had too few staff, (very occasionally too many), to meet the demands it faces. It feels like workforce crisis has followed workforce crisis. Meeting the workforce challenge is not simply a case of recruiting and training more staff or reducing demand for services through health promotion and addressing health inequalities, important as both of these obviously are. It is also a question of reducing turnover, improving productivity, devising new ways of working, maximising the potential of technology and also ensuring that the contribution of the whole NHS workforce including support workers.

Around one in four of the NHS clinical workforce work are employed in a support role. They work as Healthcare Assistants, Maternity Support Workers, Therapy Assistants, Radiography Clinical Support Workers, Assistant Practitioners, Mammography Associates and in many, more roles. This book has been framed by an understanding of the issues this workforce can face (along with what can be done to overcome these and the potential benefits of doing so). Support workers have – and continue to be – neglected. The word 'invisible' has been used by a number of researchers, think tanks and Camilla Cavendish to describe how this important workforce, who provide the bulk of face-to-face contact in many settings, are treated.

What lies at the core of this is a problem, it seems to me, a problem that has bedevilled the NHS since its creation – its failure to treat its workforce as one. This is a serious and enduring failure that has led to registered staff having clear progression pathways, status, and access to education, but support workers with little of this. Of course, this is a simplification and registered staff also face issues such as parity of esteem between for example nurses and doctors; however this is more a question of degree. The great divide between registered and support staff is much more fundamental for all the islands of excellence that exist.

Why does the NHS not, for instance, plan, and deliver a workforce approach for the nursing workforce as a whole? An approach that acknowledges that some of the nursing workforce are registered and some are not, but all of whom provide nursing care and support to patients? Instead, we have targets to recruit nurses and isolated policy developments such as the Nursing Associate, rather than a single workforce strategy. The same is true of other professions. Everyone loses by this 'two workforces' approach. Busy registered staff do not get the support they need, support workers are not able to realise their potential and service-user outcomes are not as good as they could be. There is an urgent need for the NHS to stop thinking in this way, to close the divide and think in terms of one workforce. This will go some way, perhaps a long way, to building the capacity and capability it needs to meet service demand. Doing this, though, will require a much more concentrated approach nationally and locally to support worker on-boarding, management, appraisals, learning, integration into teams and career pathways.

A one workforce approach means looking inwards and addressing the inconsistencies that support workers face with more standardisation so that everyone is clear about their scope of practice and are paid fairly and equitably for the work they do – something that is not always the case now.

Thinking and acting as one NHS workforce will help staff – who want and are able too – progress their careers from entry-level to advanced practice. For many support workers who wish to become radiographers, midwives, nurses, occupational therapists, doctors, clinical scientists or dieticians it is far too often the case that the NHS career ladder for them stops after the second or third run. A one workforce approach, though, will also mean that those who do not want to leave support roles (most of the workforce) will have rewarding careers.

The fact that the NHS does not think of its employees in these ways, and some of its employees do not either, is a product of its history. The evolution of support roles has so often been in the shadow of the development of registered staff and moves to close the professions. This has meant that support workers have been defined by what they cannot do rather than what they can, as subordinate, on occasions even as a threat to registered staff or as a stalking horse for local pay bargaining, cuts and de-skilling. It is only in recent years that they are being more explicitly thought about in terms of what they can do and what they can contribute to care.

Things are changing for the better, but it is still left, for example, to individual employers to decide what qualifications and experience new recruits should possess meaning NHS trusts located next to each other can ask for very different recruitments for the same role, which they probably describe differently as well. The development of national education and competency frameworks is very welcome albeit with the caveat that they are not mandatory. The future could see a support worker working in Truo able to perform the same tasks, underpinned by occupationally relevant qualifications, as one working in Taunton, Telford or Torbay. They might even have the same job description and title. Standardisation and consistency were the key changes Camilla Cavendish called for.

There is no excuse for this not to happen. All that is needed is there and the main thing that is needed is for the NHS to think of its workforce as one workforce.

References

Cavendish, C. (2013). *Cavendish Review. An Independent Enquiry into Healthcare Assistants and Support Workers in the NHS and Social Care Settings.* London, Department of Health. Available from: https://assets.publishing.service.gov.uk/government/uploads/system/uploads/attachment_data/file/236212/Cavendish_Review.pdf

Palinkas, L. A., Horwitz, S. M., Green, C. A., Wisdom, J. P., Duan, N., and Hoagwood, K. (2015). Purposeful sampling for qualitative data collection and analysis in mixed method implementation research. *Administration and Policy in Mental Health* 42(5), 533–544. https://doi.org/10.1007/s10488-013-0528-y

INDEX

Printed in the United States
by Baker & Taylor Publisher Services